# PRACTICAL USE OF

# HOMEOPATHIC
# MEDICINES

Produced by Bookmaker

Original title: HOMEOPATHIE - LE CONSEIL AU QUOTIDIEN
© Boiron France, 1996    ISBN 2- 85742-129-X

Graphic design by CEGEP
Desktop publication by Imprimerie Brailly
Cover design by Bernard Flageul
Cover painting: *Avec titre* by Jean-Philippe Aubanel, 1996 - Photo by Didier Michalet

Translated by Anne-Marie Cervera and Graham Fox

*Special thanks to Bonnie Price Lofton for her help*

© BOIRON 2006
ISBN 978-2-85742-204-0

# PRACTICAL USE OF
# HOMEOPATHIC
# MEDICINES

**Michèle BOIRON**
Pharmacist

**Alain PAYRE-FICOT**
Pharmacist

EDITIONS BOIRON

# TABLE OF CONTENTS

# FOREWORD

On OPENING THIS BOOK, some readers may be thinking: "*yet another work on homeopathic counseling for pharmacists*". This is indeed true, but in my view, it is all for the best. Each work in this domain has its own originality, its own specific character. The present publication is the result of the close and careful collaboration of two very experienced dispensing pharmacists.

My daughter, Michèle, has always been "steeped" in homeopathy, in all senses of the word. It helped her get over the illnesses and mishaps of childhood, so she has been able to observe its efficacy for herself. She has also lived in a family where every day represented an ongoing drive to improve and promote the production technology, standardization and control of the medicines, the research demonstrating their pharmacodynamic efficacy, and the regulatory framework necessary to accompany their preparation and to give homeopathy an official status in France.

As for our colleague and friend Alain Payre-Ficot, he decided some years ago that he wished to be better prepared to respond to the desires of his customers, and he began to study homeopathy with great enthusiasm. Over the years, impressed by the daily evidence of the efficacy of this approach, he has considerably developed the homeopathic aspect of his activity.

This book is the sum of their combined practical experience, and is thus of great value as a reflection of their competence and their pragmatism.

For my part, I am convinced that no effort must be spared in our determination to enlighten and inform our fellow dispensing pharmacists of the various aspects of homeopathy. If homeopathy now has an exceptional standing in France, it is thanks to them. In the space of a few years they have come from a general lack of knowledge on the subject to an exact recognition of the usefulness of homeopathic medicines prepared in rigorous accordance with Good Manufacturing Practices.

The great majority of these pharmacists, driven by a strong sense of professional responsibility, have followed specialized university courses. They have thus become not simply retailers of homeopathic medicines, but qualified medical providers who can draw on a firm basis of knowledge. These efforts are particularly praiseworthy, as the training involved adds yet another charge to the countless responsibilities of dispensing pharmacists.

Today, when the economics of health care are increasingly scrutinized, and when the iatrogenic effects of certain medicines is of increasing concern, it seems to me essential that dispensing pharmacists should include homeopathic medicines in their advice to their customers, with competence and without dogmatism.

I urge all my colleagues to read this work, which will provide them with effective help and an added dimension in their daily practice.

*JEAN BOIRON*
*(1906-1996)*

*This foreword is the last text written by Jean Boiron, on July 10th 1996. It shows the remarkable passion of a man who worked throughout his professional life for the scientific recognition of homeopathy, in particular through the development of research and teaching.*
*It also shows the complete trust he placed in dispensing pharmacists for their role in this development; having begun his professional life as a dispensing pharmacist, he fully understood the importance and the key role they play in the health care network.*
*We would like to take this opportunity to pay homage to the exceptional personality of this pioneer, and to express our admiration and our gratitude.*

# PREFACE

IT IS A PARTICULAR PLEASURE for me to introduce this work by Michèle Boiron and Alain Payre-Ficot, two pharmacists who both have a passionate interest in homeopathy.

In 1976, together with Professor Georges Netien (then holder of the Chair in Botany, and now Honorary Professor of the Faculty of Pharmacy of Lyon), we created a university diploma in homeopathy. This was the first diploma of its type to be awarded by a French university; since then, others have followed:

• Lille
• Aix-Marseille
• Bordeaux
• Dijon
• Limoges
• Nantes
• Poitiers
• Toulouse

The first students to follow this course, graduating in June 1977, included a large proportion of dispensing pharmacists who had already been practicing for some years; among them were the authors of the present work.

Since then, we have had numerous occasions to appreciate the high level of competence in homeopathy of both the authors. Today, Michèle Boiron devotes one morning each week to teaching homeopathic counseling on the diploma course.

**This book, written by health care professionals for health care professionals, has been produced for you, physicians, nurses, dispensing pharmacists and students, in order to facilitate the integration of homeopathy into your daily practice.**

As pharmacists occupy a strategic position between doctor and patient, they will often be called on for this sort of advice. They must thus have an adequate level of competence in homeopathy. They must also realize that customers interested in homeopathy will be more demanding, will be likely to try self-medication, will be inclined to ask questions (often very pertinent ones), and will frequently consult books on homeopathy. Prescribing nurses and physicians are also increasingly asked for the natural, simple and safe resources of homeopathy.

Consulting a homeopathic materia medica can be a lengthy process. It presupposes a sound knowledge of homeopathy and can appear daunting to a person who has never undergone a specific training in this domain.

The authors have clearly understood this problem, and offer the reader the benefit of their experience in a series of clear and straightforward entries on different aspects of homeopathic therapeutics, which are accessible to a non-specialist health care professional. This "user-friendly" presentation, completed by a summary in table form, will enable a medicine to be chosen rapidly, corresponding to a definite key symptom, or on the basis of one or more reported symptoms, or for a particular disease or disorder.

The medicine recommended may be "single", but the pharmacist may also choose to propose one of the many special complex medicines available. A combination of homeopathic and allopathic recommendations is also envisaged; the authors indicate the limits to be respected in such cases, and always advise that a qualified physician be consulted whenever this seems necessary.

Pharmacists must also be capable of explaining the prescription of a homeopathic physician; they should be able to understand the choice of dilutions prescribed, and to distinguish the constitutional medicine from the various functional medicines.

Explaining a prescription requires a sound knowledge of the homeopathic materia medica. For this, the user can refer to the second part of the book, where the major polychrests (key medicines with a wide range of applications) and the other medicines cited in the section on therapeutics are all dealt with. Making good use of the materia medica is more problematic than consulting the entries in the previous section, and presupposes that the reader has already acquired a sense of the particular reasoning inherent in a homeopathic approach.

To conclude, we can affirm that, thanks to Michèle Boiron and Alain Payre-Ficot, pharmacists, prescribing nurses and physicians now have at their disposal a work written in clear and precise language, without superfluous commentary, which will give them valuable assistance in offering speedy and effective advice in the course of their daily practice.

*Professor Jean Raynaud*

# Introduction

*This introduction has been written for French Pharmacists. In France, not only patients will likely seek advice and counsel from their community pharmacist about their health concerns, but a large proportion of medicines recommended by pharmacists are homeopathic medicines. This just shows how homeopathy can be easily integrated in the daily practice of pharmacists, but also nurses, physicians, and many other health care professionals, for the benefit of their patients. This book provides a precise and quick reference to busy doctors, nurses and pharmacists of any country where homeopathic medicines are available. Most of the warnings apply to all types of health care professionals. In the United States, homeopathic medicines have been regulated as drugs by the Food and Drug Administration since 1938.*

*(Note from the Editor)*

EVERY DAY IN THE WORK OF A FRENCH DISPENSING PHARMACIST, **homeopathy** takes up time and space and calls for knowledgeable intervention, yet there may well be neither the time nor the desire to consult those works which might be of assistance in this domain.

We are **pharmacists**, and like all our colleagues, at each moment in our professional lives we have to deal with customers who are also patients. In France, 39% of these customers use homeopathy regularly and another 32% say they would be willing to do so! Approximately 25,000 French doctors, both general practitioners and specialists, prescribe this form of treatment. A poll conducted a few years ago showed that 70% of French general practitioners found homeopathy to be effective. This shows that homeopathic medicine would seem to be set to play an increasingly important role in health care.

According to a study conducted in June 1996, 67% of French dispensing pharmacists consider homeopathy to be a form of therapy which is both medical and scientific.

In addition, it offers a real and exciting opportunity to recommend treatments that are both effective and in keeping with the demands of our customers. It enhances our role as "health advisers".

To this end, we must understand and learn about homeopathy, just as we have had to familiarize ourselves with all the other therapeutic approaches. Homeopathy has its own specific features and requirements, which is only to be expected. All the same, it is now quite clear that one does not have to "believe in it for it to work"! That particular cliché can now be shelved.

**The primary role of the pharmacist is first of all to ensure that customers know how to make the best use of homeopathic medicines.** We should not forget that 80% of these customers come to us with a prescription. It is thus absolutely necessary that the patient be clearly informed concerning the following points, which may seem obvious but are not always so to a patient new to homeopathy:
- **multi-dose tubes of pellets:** the dosage indicated by the physician must be respected (i.e. the number of pellets to be taken each

time, generally 5), and the pellets should not be touched, for hygienic reasons;
- **unit-dose tubes:** (smaller tubes containing small pellets): the entire contents of the unit-dose tube must be taken each time.

As to the timing of the doses, all homeopathic medicines are to be taken some distance away from meals (15 minutes before, or half an hour after).

**As for those customers who come to us for advice, it has to be admitted that it is rare for them to request a homeopathic medicine spontaneously. So, why should homeopathy be recommended?**

First of all, your own experience will tend to lead you in this direction: you will quickly observe the efficacy of homeopathy, and you will soon find yourself wanting to recommend it without hesitation.

In addition, homeopathy has no side effects; in this respect, it has a great advantage over most other medicines, in particular when the treatment is for an infant, an expectant or nursing mother, an elderly person already taking numerous other medicines, or indeed for a sportsman or sportswoman, or for a student. Each year in France, 50,000 prescriptions for tranquilizers are delivered for babies less than nine months old, and 400,000 for children under seven; would it not be wiser, as a first line of treatment, to try homeopathy?

Although homeopathy has been officially recognized in France since 1965, it still draws ironic smiles from those who remain ignorant (sometimes deliberately) of the **scientific studies carried out by independent research laboratories** throughout the world, which have been published in leading medical journals. These results are no longer ignored by medical specialists, however. Some examples include:

- the publications of Prof. Bonavida (University of California, Los Angeles) on dilutions of tumorous cells;
- the publications of Prof. Doutremepuich (laboratory of hematology of the University of Bordeaux), showing the activity of dilutions of aspirin on the formation of blood clots.

Clinically, numerous double blind trials have produced positive results, some of them being published in prestigious medical journals such as **The Lancet** or **Pediatrics.** These include the works of Dr Reilly (University of Glasgow) on respiratory allergies, those of Dr Jacobs (Seattle) on acute gastroenteritis in children in Nicaragua, and those of Dr Fisher in the field of rheumatology. An increasing number of hospitals are opening their doors to homeopathic doctors to work in services dealing with serious conditions such as AIDS and cancer, with the aim of integrating homeopathy into a more global approach to patient care.

We have come a long way since the earlier days of research, such as the work carried out by Jean Boiron and Lise Wurmser on *Arsenicum album* at the beginning of the 1960s!

**Before using this book, which is designed to serve as a guide giving practical help and assistance, we would like the reader to bear clearly in mind the two golden rules of homeopathic advice in the pharmacy.**

1. The pharmacist's advice should only seek to address the symptoms of an occasional condition in the patient. If the symptoms become repetitive or chronic, a homeopathic physician must be consulted.

2. The pharmacist's advice must be limited in time. Patients should be informed that if no improvement is experienced within 48 hours, it is **essential** that they consult their physician.

# Definition and history

## Definition of homeopathy

Homeopathy is a system of therapeutics based on two fundamental notions:
- the phenomenon of similars;
- the infinitesimal dose.

The basic principle of modern homeopathy can be set out as follows:

*"Any pharmacologically active substance, capable of provoking certain symptoms in a healthy individual when administered in weight doses, can eliminate similar symptoms in a sick person, if it is used in a very low dosage."*

This observation, first made and subsequently renewed by Hahnemann, had already been expressed in less precise terms by Hippocrates, who declared that *"like cures like"*.

The story of Hahnemann's life illuminates this discovery.

Samuel Hahnemann, born in 1755 in Meissen in Saxony, was a German physician specialized in toxicology and pharmacology; he began his medical practice at the age of 24. He was soon disappointed by the absence of effective therapeutic results and by the limitations of the medicine practiced in his time (he considered the drugs in general use to be too aggressive), and he decided to cease practicing. In order to earn his living, he translated various works until one day, when reading the materia medica of the Scottish doctor William Cullen, he was confused by the explanation given of the action of quinine, commonly used to treat "swamp fever". He thus decided to experiment on himself and on members of his entourage, so as to determine the real effects of quinine.

## Hahnemann's discovery

Hahnemann, who was in good health at the time, observed that a low dose of quinine gave him a fever, which was altogether comparable to the swamp fever (malaria) counteracted by the same quinine administered in weight doses.

## Hahnemann's hypothesis

Reversing his empirical observations, Hahnemann conceived of the possibility of curing malarial patients with small doses of quinine. He thus set forth the following hypothesis:

**"According to the dosage employed, would it not be possible for the same substance to be capable of provoking symptoms in a healthy individual and suppressing**

similar symptoms in a sick individual?"

In order to verify this hypothesis, Hahnemann undertook a systematic testing (or "proving") of the pharmacological substances of his time on healthy individuals, in order to determine, as he wrote, the "pure effects" of these substances.

The collection of data thus gathered concerning each of these drugs constitutes the pathogenesis of the drug in question.

Hahnemann eliminated all the compound remedies used at the time, which were based on a mixture of substances, and administered only single drugs in varying dosages. He first conducted these trials on himself, his family and friends, and then on patients, using small doses of substances which, when given in larger doses, produce in a healthy human the same symptoms as those observed in the patient.

He noticed that there was an aggravation, often only temporary, on starting the treatment, and he thus reduced the quantity of the substance administered: this is the origin of the scale of successive dilutions.

He realized that these dilutions, far from reducing the therapeutic efficacy, actually reinforced it, on condition that a vigorous agitation was carried out between each dilution (a process which Hahnemann called "dynamization"). Clinical confirmation was provided by the observation that the majority of the patients were cured.

Hahnemann's success brought him fame and international recognition. Homeopathy developed fast, but Hahnemann soon found himself faced with hostile reactions from some doctors and pharmacists.

Hahnemann's first article was written in 1796, and he subsequently published a number of longer works, which were later translated into French and English:

1810 : *Organon der rationallen Heilkunde;*

1819 : a second edition of the *Organon der Heilkunst*, corrected and completed.

Starting in 1811, Hahnemann began publishing the results of his experiments on healthy individuals. He enriched his own work with that of his students, and in 1821 published his *Materia Medica Pura* in a single volume, before adding a second part in 1834.

Twelve years of experimentation were necessary for Hahnemann's hypothesis to be fully embodied in a confirmed and definable method of treatment, based on the principle (or "law") of similars.

**"Any sick individual can be cured by means of small dynamized doses of the substance which, when given in stronger doses to a healthy individual, provokes the same symptoms as those presented by the patient."**

Defining homeopathy by the popular notion of "the disease curing the disease" is of course an erroneous over-simplification, but it nevertheless carries within it the key principle that **"like cures like"** (Greek *homoios*, 'like' + *pathos*, 'suffering').

# What is a pathogenesis?

A pathogenesis is the collection of symptoms observed in a healthy human in the course of the accidental or experimental administration of a pharmacologically active substance, in a measurable weight dose.

### Intoxication

*a) Acute intoxication* displays a number of characteristic symptoms: vomiting, diarrhea, followed by lesions which can lead to death. The signs are not specific to the substance involved.

*b) Chronic intoxication* (of occupational origin, for example) is slow and progressive, provoking a variety of symptoms which are specific to the substance in question; they are thus of greater interest to the medical researcher.

The gradual onset of the intoxication favors the development of functional symptoms, which are carefully noted.

### Experimentation on healthy individuals

This type of experimentation must be carried out using a substance which is absolutely clearly defined, and is given gradually and repeatedly in weight doses which must remain at subtoxic levels. The experiment is to be carried out on a number of subjects, known to be healthy, and chosen to constitute a representative population.

Any symptoms which appear are observed in great detail, and noted down in the terms employed by the subjects.

This experimentation on healthy humans allows the whole range of personal sensations of the subjects to be listed, as well as the modalities of the symptoms, which are essential for the physician to determine the appropriate medicine for a patient.

The pathogeneses of the various medicines are grouped together in works known as *Homeopathic Materia Medica*.

## Application of the method to the person seeking treatment

In order to understand the **principle of similars**, let us consider some examples.

A woman suffering from cystitis with hematuria, with intense burning pains before, during, and after micturition, can be cured with low doses of Spanish Fly *(Cantharis)* which, in weight doses, provokes similar symptoms and reactive modalities in a healthy individual.

A patient exhausted by constant spurting diarrhea, accompanied by cold sweats and cramping pains, can be cured by small doses of *Veratrum album*, which in larger doses causes a similar clinical picture in a healthy individual.

In his published introduction to homeopathy, Dr Rousson, a leading homeopathic physician in Lyon, gives the following account of an experiment which illustrates the application of the principle.

*"Two identical twins are suffering from frothy diarrhea with glairy mucous vomiting, after eating unripe fruit.*

*In accordance with the similarity of the symptoms, the same medicine, Ipecac, is given to both twins. But one of them is given the mother tincture and the other, Ipecac in 9C.*

*What do we notice?*

*The condition of the first twin worsens, while the second shows a marked improvement. In the first case, we can see that a 'morbid addition' has been obtained, while in the second, there is a subtraction of the pathological symptoms."*

## Prescription of the homeopathic medicine

Prescription requires a drawing together and a careful comparison of two areas of observation:

1) **the clinical picture** presented by the patient;

2) **the toxicologic picture**, resulting from the experimental administration of a substance in a healthy human.

The drug which provokes the closest symptoms is known as the "simillimum".

The greater the degree of correspondence of the two pictures, the surer the choice of medicine, which can also be prescribed in higher dilutions than when the correspondence is less clear.

It is thus vital that the physician be thoroughly familiar with the pathogeneses of the various medicines.

**The clinical picture** brings together all the symptoms observed in a patient.

These symptoms can be considered in terms of a hierarchy.

• *Local signs*: objective symptoms based on observation (bruising, warts, eczema, etc.).

• *General signs*: these are the expression of a general reactive mode (fever, cough, diarrhea, etc.).

• *Mental and psychological signs*: these should include only those modifications of the individual's habitual behavior which can be ascribed to the disease.

• *Anatomicopathological signs*: i.e. the histological symptoms.

All these symptoms, which represent the expression of the particular reaction of the patient to his or her disease, are made more specific by the circumstances in which they appear. These circumstances constitute what are known as the "**reactive modalities**": aggravation, improvement, laterality, etc.

The local and general signs are important for the choice of medicine.

Let us take the example of fever:

- high fever (102.2°F-103.1°F) of sudden onset, **with dry skin** (no sweating), indicates *Aconitum napellus*;

- high fever (102.2°F-103.1°F) of sudden onset but **with perspiration**, indicates *Belladonna*;

- continuous fever, **without thirst**, will respond to *Gelsemium sempervirens*;

- continuous fever, **accompanied by thirst**, indicates *Bryonia alba*.

The physician will attach great importance to the modality of the symptom. For example, a burning pain relieved by heat constitutes a distinctive sign calling for *Arsenicum album*, as the majority of burns are relieved by cold.

# The pharmaceutical conception of homeopathic medicines

### The infinitesimal dose

The second fundamental principle of homeopathy is the use of the medicine in highly diluted concentrations.

This basic principle, which the general public is often aware of and takes to be the main particularity of homeopathy, is in fact simply the corollary of the principle of similars.

Indeed, if the patient were given the appropriate medicine but in too strong a concentration, the disease symptoms would be aggravated.

As we have already seen in the experiments conducted by Hahnemann, the progressive diminution of the quantities of substance employed leads to the production of infinitesimal doses which only become really effective after "succussion" (prolonged shaking between each dilution), the objective of which is the dynamization of the active principle.

The current French pharmacopoeia specifies that this process of dynamization must be carried out in the pharmaceutical preparation of homeopathic medicines.

The infinitesimal dose is justified by the observation of experimental results, confirmed in clinical practice.

### The production process

Homeopathic preparations are obtained from substances of vegetable origin, or from animals (e.g. venoms), and from chemical substances, either mineral (e.g. *Cuprum metallicum* = copper) or organic (e.g. glands).

*a) Strains of vegetable origin*: the **mother tinctures** (or MT) of vegetable origin are obtained by alcoholic maceration of fresh (or less frequently, dried) plants or parts of plants. The maceration takes place in glass or stainless steel recipients, and lasts at least three weeks.

After maceration, the mother tinctures are decanted, filtered, stored in particular conditions (as regards temperature, low light, ventilation, etc.), and are rigorously monitored. The mass of mother tinture thus obtained is ten times greater than that of the primary substance (calculated in respect of the mass of this primary substance in dehydrated form).

**b) Strains of animal origin:** These are made up of a 1/20 alcoholic maceration of:
- whole live animals (e.g. *Apis mellifica* = whole bees; *Formica rufa* = red ants, etc.;)
- certain parts or organs taken from animals, or certain secretions (e.g. *Sepia* = squid ink)
- venoms (*Lachesis mutus* = venom of *Bothrops surucucu*; *Vipera* = venom of *Vipera aspis*).

**c) Strains of chemical origin**
(mineral or organic) include:
- simple or composite substances: metals, metalloids, hormones, vitamins;
- chemical complexes of natural or synthetic origin (*Natrum muriaticum, Calcarea ostreica*).

**d) Medicines obtained from:**
- products which are not chemically defined, such as serums, vaccines, toxins and toxoids, viruses, etc. (*Tuberculinum* is thus obtained from cultures of *Mycobacterium tuberculosis*);
- from pathological secretions or excretions (*Psorinum* is obtained from a lysate of serous fluid from scabies lesions);
- from pure bacterial cultures (*Colibacillinum* is a lysate obtained from cultures of *Escherichia coli*)

**Allersodes**
They are obtained from allergens such as pollen, cat hairs, household dust, acarids, cigarettes, etc.

**Hetero-Isotherapeutics**
These are homeopathic attenuations of botanical, zoological, or chemical substances which have been ingested or otherwise absorbed by the body and are believed to have produced a disease or disorder which interferes with homeostasis.
All isotherapeutics require a medical prescription.

**Dilutions**
The mother tincture or the chemical or animal strain are the starting points for the preparation of the dilutions.
Several types of dilutions are used in homeopathy.

**a) Hahnemannian centesimal dilutions (C)**
These 1/100 dilutions are the most commonly used, and are prepared by adding one part of the base substance to 99 parts of a solvent. The mixture is vigorously shaken (or "dynamized") by a vibrating device; **the first Hahnemannian centesimal dilution is thus obtained (1C). One**

part of this 1C dilution, mixed with 99 parts of solvent in a new flask and dynamized, constitutes the 2C dilution, and so on up to 30C. Thirty flasks are thus required for a 30C preparation.

The most commonly prescribed centesimal dilutions in France are 4, 5, 7, 9, 12, 15, and 30C.

## b) Hahnemannian decimal dilutions (X)

These are successive 1/10 dilutions prepared using exactly the same method as for the Hahnemannian centesimals.

The most commonly prescribed decimal dilutions are 1X, 3X, 6X.

## c) Korsakovian dilutions (CK)

In 1832, the Russian Korsakov proposed a method of dilution known as the "single flask" technique, in order to avoid the use of large numbers of different flasks.

5 mL of mother tincture are placed in a flask, which is shaken vigorously and then emptied by aspiration. This procedure leaves 1% of the initial volume in the flask. Purified water is added to dilute the traces of the mother tincture adhering to the sides of flask, the flask is shaken again, and the **first Korsakovian dilution (1CK) is thus obtained.** A repetition of the operation gives the second Korsakovian dilution, and so on.

The most commonly prescribed dilutions are 200 CK, 1,000 CK (or 1 M) and 10,000 CK (or 10 M). They are generally delivered on medical prescription.

This method thus requires a long series of operations in order to obtain the high dilutions. The preparation of Korsakovian dilutions is carried out by means of an automatic device, ensuring the precision and the repetition of the operations.

Whatever type of dilution is chosen, the operation is very delicate and must be undertaken with great precaution.

The atmosphere must be as pure as possible. Town air, even when not significantly polluted, contains traces of sulfur, mercury, and lead in suspension, which can alter the preparation by combining with the base substance during the dynamization process. This is why an air filtering system is used inside laboratories, to lower the level of pollution. Jean Boiron originated the idea of carrying out the dilution process within a "laminar flow enclosure", which filters the air so as to obtain less than 100 particles for 30 liters of air (class 100 of American Federal

Standard 209). The level is continuously monitored to ensure that this norm is respected.

Air purity by itself does not suffice, of course: the equipment used and the solvent must also be rigorously controlled.

- The solvent is pharmaceutical grade 70% v/v alcohol.
- The flasks used for the dilutions are washed three times in succession in demineralized water, then sterilized at 180°C for an hour. These flasks are specially shaped and made from an appropriate type of glass; before use, the ambient air inside them is extracted and replaced with purified air from the laminar flow enclosure.

## The triturations

Strains which are insoluble in water and alcohol are ground together with lactose: this process is known as trituration.

In a mortar, one part of the substance is triturated together with 99 parts of lactose; the 1C trituration is thus obtained. The operation is then renewed in a second mortar using one part of the 1C trituration, so as to produce the 2C; a third operation gives the 3C. With this 3C trituration, still in the form of a lactose powder, a liquid dilution can be obtained by dissolving one part of the trituration in 99 parts of solvent (purified water or alcohol in various titers); the 4C dilution is thus obtained as a liquid, which can then be subjected to a series of dilutions. This solubility starting at the 3C trituration, which was accepted by Hahnemann, is now recognized as being scientifically correct.

## The pellets

These are small spheres made up of a mixture of saccharose sucrose and lactose. The coating process is carried out in turbines, specially designed to operate continuously. The fabrication of small pellets (200 per gram) takes about two weeks; several additional days are required to prepare the large pellets (20 per gram).

These neutral pellets, small and large, are transformed into medicines by impregnation with a dilution. The impregnation of the pellets was formerly performed in a single operation, and was thus only superficial, which explains why it was not recommended to touch the pellets with the fingers.

In 1961, a process of triple impregnation was perfected, allowing a deeper penetration of the sphere to be achieved, with a correspondingly more homogenous distribution of the dilution.

These two pharmaceutical forms, small and large pellets, are specific to homeopathy.

- The large pellets, presented in 4 gram tubes containing 80 pellets, are prepared in all the dilutions.
- The small pellets are presented in a unit-dose tube of 1 gram which contains about 200 small pellets. The dose should be taken all at once, allowing the small pellets to dissolve gradually under the tongue.

Other forms are also common, such as:

- drops; the excipient is 30% v/v alcohol. They are generally reserved for the low dilutions (X and mother tinctures), or for complex medicines. They are to be taken either pure, or diluted in a little water.

All the other pharmaceutical forms also exist in homeopathy: ointments, eye-drops, ampules, suppositories, pessaries, etc.

The medicines can be:

- **single**, i.e. consisting of a single active ingredient; or
- **complex**, if they are made up of a mixture of single homeopathic medicines with complementary indications.

We can thus give the following definition of the homeopathic medicine: **a homeopathic medicine is made up of one or more substances 1) which are active when administered in an infinitesimal dose, and 2) which have undergone a series of successive dilution and dynamization.**

## Particular precautions concerning storage and use of homeopathic medicines

Because of their particular diluted nature, homeopathic medicines can be affected by certain volatile substances such as camphor and perfumes.

In addition, the tubes of pellets should not be subjected to excessively high temperatures (> 115°F), as this may modify the therapeutic action of the medicine.

## Dosage and instructions for use

Homeopathic medicines should preferably be taken away from

meals (15 minutes before or 30 minutes after).

The choice of the form depends on how and when the medicine is to be used: repeated doses during the day, or one single daily, weekly or monthly dose. Ease of use for the patient should be aimed at.

The **unit-dose tube** is particularly suitable for a single dose, or for doses to be taken at widely spaced intervals.

The **multi-dose tube** containing large pellets is convenient to carry around if the medicine has to be taken repeatedly during the day.

It is recognized that the frequency of administration of the medicines depends partly on the degree of dilution.

- **The low (4C/5C/6C) or medium (7C/9C/12C) dilutions** have a action which is limited in time; they correspond to local or general symptoms and are generally administered two or three times a day until the symptoms disappear, particularly in acute cases.

- **The high dilutions (15C/30C)** are generally used for chronic conditions and for particular sensitive types; they are thus usually prescribed by the physician to be taken once a week or once every two weeks.

Contrary to received opinion, mint and coffee, if taken some time away from the medicines, do not act as antidotes. In addition, it should be made clear that homeopathic medicines are not incompatible with other types of medication, in particular with allopathic medicines, since their action is not situated on the same level. Indeed, homeopathic medicines can often work synergistically with allopathic ones.

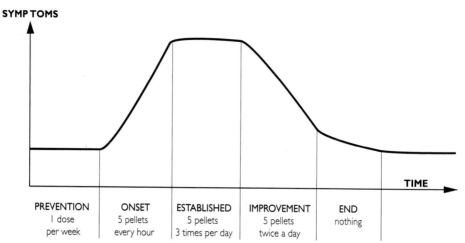

SYMPTOMS

| PREVENTION | ONSET | ESTABLISHED | IMPROVEMENT | END |
|---|---|---|---|---|
| 1 dose per week | 5 pellets every hour | 5 pellets 3 times per day | 5 pellets twice a day | nothing |

# Conclusion

Homeopathy does not cure all diseases, but it has the advantage of considering the patient as a unique entity.

Some of the products or specialties mentioned in this book may not be available in certain countries as they have not yet been registered.

# THERAPEUTICS

# ACUTE CORYZA (COMMON COLD)

Acute coryza, or common cold, is a benign condition occurring following a chill.

It is characterized by the appearance of nasal obstruction with or without discharge. Sneezing is common.

## DETERMINING SYMPTOMS

Acute coryza is likely to be contracted when there are marked variations in temperature or seasonal changes.

It may have an epidemic character, during periods when influenza is prevalent.

Coryza may be accompanied by:
- fever,
- headache,
- loss of taste,
- loss of smell.

A cold which is not attended to "settle in the chest", and give rise to coughing.

Coryza can be classified in two main forms:
- dry coryza,
- wet coryza.

## PRINCIPAL MEDICINES

### DRY CORYZA

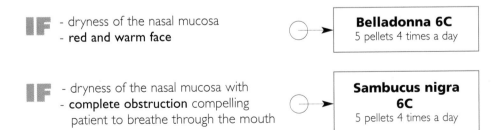

**IF**
- dryness of the nasal mucosa
- **red and warm face**

→ **Belladonna 6C**
5 pellets 4 times a day

**IF**
- dryness of the nasal mucosa with
- **complete obstruction** compelling patient to breathe through the mouth

→ **Sambucus nigra 6C**
5 pellets 4 times a day

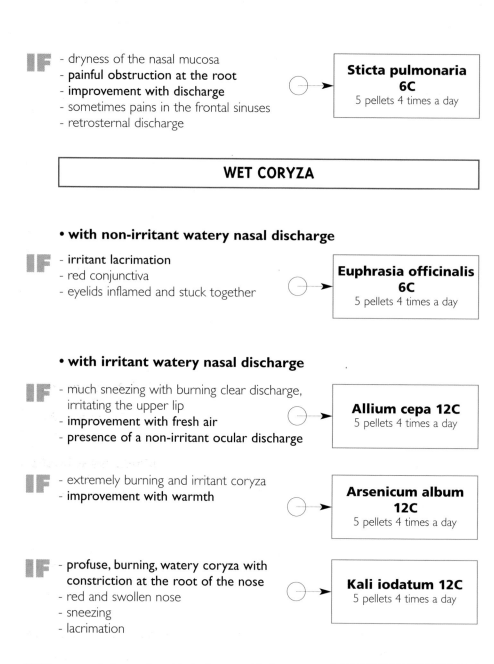

**IF**
- dryness of the nasal mucosa
- **painful obstruction at the root**
- **improvement with discharge**
- sometimes pains in the frontal sinuses
- retrosternal discharge

**Sticta pulmonaria
6C**
5 pellets 4 times a day

## WET CORYZA

### • with non-irritant watery nasal discharge

**IF**
- irritant lacrimation
- red conjunctiva
- eyelids inflamed and stuck together

**Euphrasia officinalis
6C**
5 pellets 4 times a day

### • with irritant watery nasal discharge

**IF**
- much sneezing with burning clear discharge, irritating the upper lip
- **improvement with fresh air**
- **presence of a non-irritant ocular discharge**

**Allium cepa 12C**
5 pellets 4 times a day

**IF**
- extremely burning and irritant coryza
- **improvement with warmth**

**Arsenicum album
12C**
5 pellets 4 times a day

**IF**
- **profuse, burning, watery coryza with constriction at the root of the nose**
- red and swollen nose
- sneezing
- lacrimation

**Kali iodatum 12C**
5 pellets 4 times a day

**IF**
- **excoriating and acrid discharge with fever**
- **shivering along the spine**
- headache like a headband round the head
- heavy eyelids
- **aches and pains**
- absence of thirst (in a context of influenza)

**Gelsemium
sempervirens 12C**
5 pellets 4 times a day

### • with thick nasal discharge

**IF**
- whitish or grayish, thick, glairy nasal discharge
- diminished hearing
- cracking in the ears when swallowing or when blowing nose

→ **Kali muriaticum 12C**
5 pellets 4 times a day

**Kali muriaticum** corresponds to the second phase of inflammation.

**IF**
- non-irritant and profuse nasal discharge, most often yellow but sometimes a homogeneous greenish-yellow
- dry nose obstructed in the evening and at night
- dry cough at night, loose in the morning
- loss of sense of taste and smell

→ **Pulsatilla 12C**
5 pellets 4 times a day

**IF**
- adhesive, very viscous, greenish-yellow nasal discharge, forming crusts in the nostrils

→ **Kali bichromicum 12C**
5 pellets 4 times a day

**IF**
- greenish-yellow, foul-smelling nasal discharge
- inflammation and ulceration of the nostrils
- hypersalivation
- tongue retaining teethmarks

→ **Mercurius solubilis 12C**
5 pellets 4 times a day

**IF**
- thick, adhesive, yellowish, viscous and thready discharge, forming plugs, with posterior nasal discharge

→ **Hydrastis canadensis 12C**
5 pellets 4 times a day

**Hydrastis canadensis 3X** promotes secretion and loosens mucus. **High** dilutions dry them up.

### • Special cases

**IF**
- coryza related to ambient humidity and cold

→ **Dulcamara 12C**
5 pellets 4 times a day

- **coryza after getting wet,**
  with sneezing, articular stiffness,
  and aching

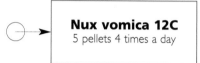

**Rhus toxicodendron 12C**
5 pellets 4 times a day

- **spasmodic sneezing in the morning**
  immediately on rising
  and during the day

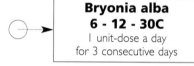

**Nux vomica 12C**
5 pellets 4 times a day

- pulmonary complications
  are to be avoided
  (coryza becoming "chesty"),
  prescribe

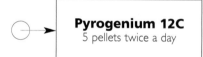

**Bryonia alba 6 - 12 - 30C**
I unit-dose a day
for 3 consecutive days

- tendency to infection

**Pyrogenium 12C**
5 pellets twice a day

## SPECIALTIES

- **COLDCALM** ® : dissolve 2 tablets in the mouth every 2 hours up to 6 times a day
- **SINUSALIA** ® : dissolve 2 tablets in the mouth every 2 hours up to 6 times a day
- **COLD CAREKIT** contains **Allium cepa 6C, Belladonna 6C** and **Kali bichromicum 6C**
- **SINUS CAREKIT** contains **Hepar Sulphuris calcareum 30C, Kali bichromicum 6C** and **Mezereum 6C**

# ACUTE CORYZA

## DRY CORYZA

- **Belladonna 6C**
  - dryness of mucous membranes
  - "tumor - rubor - dolor - calor"

- **Sambucus nigra 6C**
  - total nasal obstruction

- **Sticta pulmonaria 6C**
  - sensation of painful obstruction at the root of the nose
  - urge to blow nose with no result
  - improvement when discharge starts

## WET CORYZA

### NON-IRRITANT WATERY NASAL DISCHARGE

- **Euphrasia officinalis 6C**
  - non-irritant watery nasal discharge
  - irritant lacrimation

### IRRITANT WATERY NASAL DISCHARGE

- **Allium cepa 12C**
  - watery nasal discharge irritating the upper lip
  - improvement with fresh air
  - non-irritant lacrimation

- **Arsenicum album 12C**
  - very irritant and intensely burning nasal discharge
  - improvement with warmth

- **Kali iodatum 12C**
  - profuse burning watery discharge
  - constriction at the root of the nose
  - swollen red nose

- **Gelsemium sempervirens 12C**
  - excoriating discharge
  - fever and shivering
  - headache
  - pains and aches

### THICK NASAL DISCHARGE

- **Kali muriaticum 12C**
  - thick whitish discharge
  - diminished hearing
  - cracking in the ears when swallowing or when blowing nose

- **Pulsatilla 12C**
  - discharge most often yellow, sometimes green
  - dry nose obstructed at night
  - cough dry at night, loose cough during the day
  - loss of taste and smell

- **Kali bichromicum 12C**
  - adhesive, viscous, greenish-yellow discharge forming crusts in the nostrils

- **Mercurius solubilis 12C**
  - greenish-yellow nasal discharge with a foul smell
  - inflammation and ulceration of nostrils
  - tongue keeping imprint of teeth
  - hypersalivation

- **Hydrastis canadensis 12C**
  - adhesive, viscous, thready, yellowish discharge, forming plugs with posterior nasal discharge

- **Hydrastis canadensis 3X**
  - promotes secretions and loosens mucus, whereas higher dilutions dry them up

### SPECIAL CASES

- **Dulcamara 12C**
  - coryza related to ambient humidity and cold

- **Rhus toxicodendron 12C**
  - coryza after getting wet, with articular stiffness
  - aches and pains
  - sneezing

- **Nux vomica 12C**
  - spasmodic sneezing immediately on rising

- **Bryonia alba 9-12-15-30C**
  - 1 unit-dose a day for 4 consecutive days if coryza becomes "chesty" (beginning of dry cough)

- **Pyrogenium 12C**
  - when infection is present

# APHONIA - HOARSENESS

Partial or total loss of the voice, in an etiological context of chill, ingestion of icy drinks, or prolonged vocal strain.

## DETERMINING SYMPTOMS

To be noted:
- etiology;
- concomitant cough;
- modified tone of voice.

## PRINCIPAL MEDICINES

**IF**
- hoarseness with croupy cough after
  exposure to dry cold wind
- with anxiety
- **absence of perspiration**

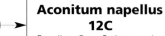

**Aconitum napellus
12C**
5 pellets 2 or 3 times a day

**IF**
- hoarseness and dryness of the larynx
- painful swallowing
- dry cough
- red face
- headache
- **perspiration**
- "tumor - rubor - dolor - calor"

**Belladonna 12C**
5 pellets 2 or 3 times a day

**IF**
- hoarseness **after getting wet** (sweating
  from exertion or rain)
- **morning hoarseness with progressive
  improvement, but aggravation towards
  the end of the day**

**Rhus toxicodendron
12C**
5 pellets 2 or 3 times a day

**IF**
- hoarseness due to paralysis of vocal cords
- **burning and rasping sensation
  in the larynx**
- improvement with warmth
- aggravation from dry cold

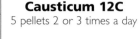

**Causticum 12C**
5 pellets 2 or 3 times a day

- hoarseness with **constantly changing tone of voice**
- rough or **bitonal** voice
- small bits of skin on the lips that the patient picks at, causing bleeding

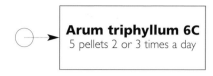

**Arum triphyllum 6C**
5 pellets 2 or 3 times a day

- hoarseness with marked **dryness** of the larynx and vocal cords
- rough voice
- burning pains when speaking

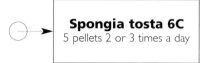

**Spongia tosta 6C**
5 pellets 2 or 3 times a day

- hoarseness from prolonged or excessive use of vocal cords (singers, orators, football fans!)

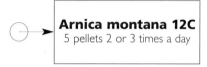

**Arnica montana 12C**
5 pellets 2 or 3 times a day

## SPECIALTY

- **ROXALIA** ® : Adults and children 12 and over : dissolve 2 tablets in the mouth every 2 hours up to 6 times a day. Children under 12: ask a doctor.

## APHONIA - HOARSENESS

- **Aconitum napellus 12C**
  - after exposure to dry cold wind
  - anxiety
  - absence of perspiration

- **Belladonna 12C**
  - dryness of larynx
  - "tumor - rubor - dolor - calor"
  - presence of sweating

- **Rhus toxicodendron 12C**
  - after rain or sweating from exertion
  - progressive improvement when starting to speak, but aggravation towards end of day

- **Causticum 12C**
  - burning and rasping sensation in the larynx
  - dry cough
  - improvement with warmth

- **Arum triphyllum 6C**
  - constantly changing tone of voice
  - small bits of skin on the lips

- **Spongia tosta 6C**
  - dryness of larynx and vocal cords
  - rough voice
  - burning pains when speaking

- **Arnica montana 12C**
  - after prolonged or excessive use of vocal cords: singers, orators, football fans

# BREAST-FEEDING

Breast-feeding mothers sometimes have problems with the quantity or quality of the milk.

In addition, in order to avoid chapping and fissuring, the mother should clean the nipples after each feeding with a mixture of equal parts of rubbing alcohol and glycerin, and should smear them each evening using an ointment with **Castor equi.**

## PRINCIPAL MEDICINES

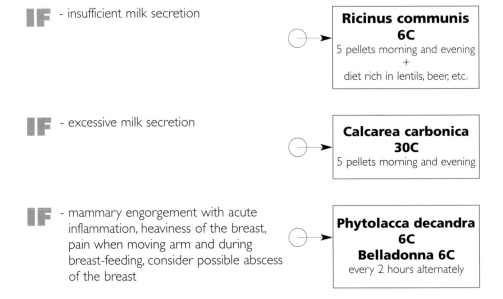

**IF** - insufficient milk secretion

> **Ricinus communis 6C**
> 5 pellets morning and evening
> +
> diet rich in lentils, beer, etc.

**IF** - excessive milk secretion

> **Calcarea carbonica 30C**
> 5 pellets morning and evening

**IF** - mammary engorgement with acute inflammation, heaviness of the breast, pain when moving arm and during breast-feeding, consider possible abscess of the breast

> **Phytolacca decandra 6C**
> **Belladonna 6C**
> every 2 hours alternately

✔ If the situation does not improve rapidly in the next 24 to 48 hours, refer to the physician.

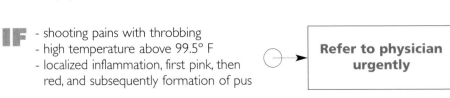

**IF** - shooting pains with throbbing
- high temperature above 99.5° F
- localized inflammation, first pink, then red, and subsequently formation of pus

> **Refer to physician urgently**

- weaning

To help with drying up secretion,
tight bandaging of the breasts is efficient

> **Calcarea carbonica 30C**
> **Pulsatilla 30C**
> **Lac caninum 30C**
> 5 pellets of each alternately every 2 hours
> **Ricinus communis 30C**
> 1 unit-dose
> on 3 consecutive mornings

---

## BREAST-FEEDING

- **Ricinus communis 6C**
  - insufficient milk secretion

- **Calcarea carbonica 30C**
  - excessive milk production

- **Phytolacca decandra 6C**
  **+ Belladonna 6C**
  - mammary engorgement with acute inflammation
  - pain when moving arm

- **Calcarea carbonica 30C**
  **+ Pulsatilla 30C**
  **+ Lac caninum 30C**
  - 5 pellets of each alternately every 2 hours, to dry up secretion when weaning
  **+ Ricinus communis 30C**
  - 1 unit- dose on 3 consecutive mornings

# BURNS SUNBURNS

Burning of the skin by heat, fire, or chemical agents.
The severity of the burn depends on the following:
- extent,
- intensity,
- age of the patient,
- localization.
The major danger of burns is **infection**.

## PRINCIPAL MEDICINES

### FIRST-DEGREE BURNS

**IF** - **pinkish skin**, stinging pains, edema, improvement with applications of cold water

**Apis mellifica 12C**
5 pellets every 2 hours

**IF** - **red skin**, burning, giving off heat

**Belladonna 6C**
5 pellets every 2 hours

### SECOND-DEGREE BURNS WITH PHLYCTENA

While waiting for the doctor:

**IF** - **large vesicles**, filled with a serous liquid, painful

**Cantharis 6C**
5 pellets 3 times a day

**IF** - **risk of infection**

**Pyrogenium 12C**
5 pellets twice a day

## SPECIALTIES

- **CALENDULA OINTMENT**: apply a thin layer, once or twice a day or as needed

or **CALENDULA LOTION**: apply 2 or 3 times a day

## BURNS - SUNBURNS

### FIRST-DEGREE BURNS

- Apis mellifica 12C
- Belladonna 6C

### SECOND-DEGREE BURNS

- Cantharis 6C
- Pyrogenium 12C

# CANKER SORES (APHTAEOUS ULCERS)

Canker sores, or aphtaeous ulcers, are small ulcerations of the oral mucosa which develop from vesicles, and which cause difficulty chewing and are painful when certain foods are ingested (particularly acidic food or drinks).

They often indicate a general inflammation of the whole digestive tract.

Their development is often favored by an excess of acidity, by eating such foods as certain berries, Swiss cheese, and walnuts, and by antibiotic medication (candidiasis).

## DETERMINING SYMPTOMS

Essentially visual.

## PRINCIPAL MEDICINES

**IF** - red vesicles located on the tongue or inside the cheeks, very painful on contact with acidic or salty foods

**Borax 6C**
5 pellets 2 or 3 times a day

**IF** - ulcerations covered with a grayish membrane

**Mercurius cyanatus 6C**
5 pellets 2 or 3 times a day

**IF** - ulcerative and necrotic tendency with intense burning

**Cantharis 6C**
5 pellets 2 or 3 times a day

**IF** - Canker sores as if stamped out with a hole-punch

**Kali bichromicum 6C**
5 pellets 2 or 3 times a day

**IF** - oral moniliasis (Candidiasis)
mouthwash with diluted bicarbonate
of soda (to alkalinize the medium)
same treatment for vaginal moniliasis,
as a complement to conventional topical treatment;
avoid using soap with an acid pH

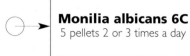

**Monilia albicans 6C**
5 pellets 2 or 3 times a day

## CANKER SORES

- **Borax 6C**
  - red vesicles on the tongue
    or inside of cheeks
  - very painful on contact
    with acidic foods

- **Mercurius cyanatus 6C**
  - ulcerations covered
    with a grayish membrane

- **Cantharis 6C**
  - ulcerative and necrotic tendency
    with intense burning

- **Kali bichromicum 6C**
  - Canker sores as if stamped out
    with a hole-punch

- **Monilia albicans 6C**
  - in case of oral moniliasis
    (as a complement to other medicines)

# CHILBLAINS

A chilblain is an inflammation localized in the extremities (hands, feet, ears, nose).
It is induced by:
- cold;
- lowing of the circulation (over-tight shoes).
Some individuals who suffer from acrocyanosis of the extremities are more sensitive **(Pulsatilla)**.

## DETERMINING SYMPTOMS

- redness and swelling
- pain
- violent itching
- possible ulceration in a second phase

## LOCAL TREATMENT

- where no ulceration: **Arnica ointment**
- where there is ulceration: **Calendula Ointment**

## PRINCIPAL MEDICINES

**IF**
- redness
- burning with itching
- tingling
- sensation of icy needles

→ **Agaricus muscarius 6C**
5 pellets 3 or 4 times a day

**IF**
- burning pain, as from red-hot needles, pinkish color
- sensitive to the slightest contact
- aggravation from heat
- aggravation at night
- improvement with cold or with cold water

→ **Apis mellifica 12C**
5 pellets 3 or 4 times a day

**IF**
- bluish or bluish-purple chilblains
- sensation of bruising
- aggravation from the slightest contact

→ **Arnica montana 12C**
5 pellets 3 or 4 times a day

**IF**
- chilblains with **intense burning**
- **improved by heat**
  or by hot applications

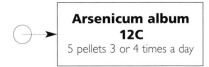

**Arsenicum album
12C**
5 pellets 3 or 4 times a day

**IF**
- **fissured**, burning chilblains
- thick skin (heels)

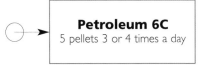

**Petroleum 6C**
5 pellets 3 or 4 times a day

**IF**
- chilblains with redness and unbearable
  **itching** at night
- **improvement with movement**

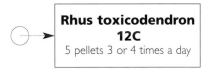

**Rhus toxicodendron
12C**
5 pellets 3 or 4 times a day

**IF**
- chilblains in an individual with **venous
  congestion,** mottled skin
- **aggravation in a warm room**
- **improvement in the open air
  and with exercise**

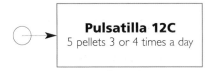

**Pulsatilla 12C**
5 pellets 3 or 4 times a day

## CHILBLAINS

- **Agaricus muscarius 6C**
  - redness, burning with itching
  - sensation of icy needles
  - improvement with warmth in bed
  - aggravation from cold

- **Apis mellifica 12C**
  - burning pains, as from red-hot needles
  - pinkish color
  - improvement with cold
  - aggravation from warmth, at night

- **Arnica montana 12C**
  - bluish or bluish-purple color
  - sensation of bruising
  - aggravation from the slightest contact

- **Arsenicum album 12C**
  - sensation of intense burning
  - improvement with heat, hot
    applications

- **Petroleum 6C**
  - sensation of burning
  - presence of fissure (heels)

- **Rhus toxicodendron 12C**
  - redness and unbearable itching at night
  - improvement with movement

- **Pulsatilla 12C**
  - venous congestion
  - mottled skin
  - improvement with exercising
    in the open air
  - aggravation in a warm room

# CONSTIPATION

Constipation is a condition of delayed bowel movements, whatever the cause.

The health care professional's role consists in:
- eliminating any possible organic cause, and intervening only in established cases of constipation, which have already been investigated;
- seeking to eliminate wrong eating habits;
- correcting dysfunction due to stress and to careless self-medication (repeated use of laxatives);
- providing the specific medicines indicated.

## DETERMINING SYMPTOMS
- frequency of bowel movements (unrelated to any medication)
- consistency of stools
- color
- presence or absence of bloating

The phenomenon of constipation does not involve only the terminal part of the intestine, but the whole of the digestive tract and the organs which play a part in digestion.

Insufficient chewing, poor gastric or pancreatic functioning, hepatobiliary dysfunction, or megacolon or dolichocolon are frequent causes of constipation.

Constipation can also be the result of poor diet or of blockages from various causes, which interfere with the reflex act of defecation:
- auto-suggestion, in patients who decide that they are unable to defecate;
- creation of a reflex action by the repeated administration of suppositories;
- blockage of transit by change of habits, travel, change or absence of activity;
- sedentary lifestyle.

## PRINCIPAL MEDICINES

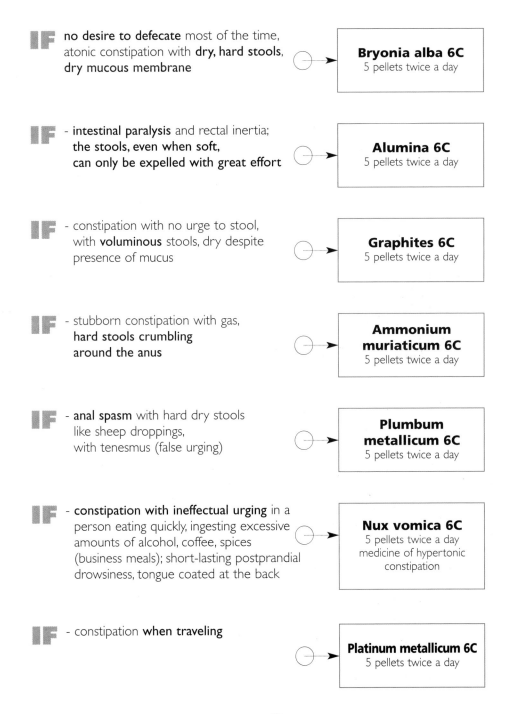

**IF** no desire to defecate most of the time, atonic constipation with **dry, hard stools**, dry mucous membrane

**Bryonia alba 6C**
5 pellets twice a day

**IF** - **intestinal paralysis** and rectal inertia; the stools, even when **soft,** can only be expelled with **great effort**

**Alumina 6C**
5 pellets twice a day

**IF** - constipation with no urge to stool, with **voluminous** stools, dry despite presence of mucus

**Graphites 6C**
5 pellets twice a day

**IF** - **stubborn constipation with gas, hard stools crumbling around the anus**

**Ammonium muriaticum 6C**
5 pellets twice a day

**IF** - **anal spasm** with hard dry stools like sheep droppings, with tenesmus (false urging)

**Plumbum metallicum 6C**
5 pellets twice a day

**IF** - **constipation with ineffectual urging** in a person eating quickly, ingesting excessive amounts of alcohol, coffee, spices (business meals); short-lasting postprandial drowsiness, tongue coated at the back

**Nux vomica 6C**
5 pellets twice a day
medicine of hypertonic constipation

**IF** - constipation **when traveling**

**Platinum metallicum 6C**
5 pellets twice a day

## CONSTIPATION

- **Bryonia alba 6C**
  - atonic constipation
  - hard dry stools

- **Alumina 6C**
  - rectal inertia + intestinal paralysis
  - soft stools, but difficult to expel

- **Graphites 6C**
  - constipation without urging
  - presence of mucus in stools

- **Ammonium muriaticum 6C**
  - hard, crumbling stools

- **Plumbum metallicum 6C**
  - "sheep droppings"
  - anal spasm

- **Nux vomica 6C**
  - constipation of "business meals"
  - ineffectual urging

- **Platinum metallicum 6C**
  - constipation when traveling

# COUGHS

Coughing is characterized principally by particular sounds, resulting from abrupt and jerky breathing. It is generally a reflex act, but may also be voluntary. It is the sign of a defensive irritation of the respiratory tract, which can involve bronchial irritation with exudative inflammation, and the formation of more or less profuse mucus which is expectorated with the coughing.

The health care professional should seek to establish:
- etiology;
- chronicity;
- accompanying symptoms affecting the general state (fever, localized pain).

A cough often follows a chill or a cold. In the initial phase, it is generally dry. As it develops, it reaches a mature phase, first without and subsequently with expectoration. If not treated, cough can clear up spontaneously, or degenerate into bronchitis. It can be the symptom of much more serious illnesses, linked to respiratory or laryngeal restriction, a permanent clearing of the throat, or a chronic morning cough. These symptoms are often less striking, and the patient becomes used to them.

**A repetitive, chronic cough definitely calls for a medical consultation.**

We are often asked to give advice in cases of coughing, and we can do so if we take account of the above considerations. Coughs can also occur in the context of an influenza epidemic, with individual reactive modalities which are often identical to those of the influenza symptoms and thus indicate the same homeopathic medicine (e.g. **Rumex crispus** if the cough is triggered by cold air, with tickling in the larynx).

## DETERMINING SYMPTOMS
Coughs are generally classified as follows:
• dry cough
• hoarse cough
• fitful cough
• loose cough

## PRINCIPAL MEDICINES

### DRY COUGH

**IF** - cough starting after exposure
to cold and dry wind with:
- high fever with sudden onset
- **absence of perspiration**
- agitation

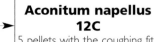

**Aconitum napellus
12C**
5 pellets with the coughing fits

**IF** - dryness of the mucous membranes with:
- high fever
- redness of the face
- **sweating**
- dejection

**Belladonna 12C**
5 pellets with the coughing fits

**IF** - **aggravation from the slightest movement**
- **improvement with immobility**
- **intense thirst**
- dryness of mucous membranes
- pain triggered by coughing

**Bryonia alba 12C**
5 pellets with the coughing fits

**IF** - constant irritation with **tickling
in the depression above the sternum**
- **aggravation from inhaling cold air**

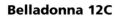

**Rumex crispus 6C**
5 pellets with the coughing fits

### HOARSE COUGH

This is a non-productive cough, characterized by a change in the tone
of the voice, which becomes deep and husky.

**IF** - dry, croupy, hoarse cough, with
wheezing and respiratory difficulty
(**noise resembling a saw cutting
through pinewood**)
- **dryness and burning of the throat**
with some degree of asphyxia
- aggravation at night around midnight,
lying with the head low
- improvement with hot drinks

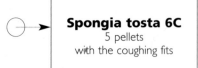

**Spongia tosta 6C**
5 pellets
with the coughing fits

**Spongia tosta** is an excellent medicine for acute laryngitis and laryngitis stridulosa. To prevent laryngitis stridulosa, it is possible to combine **Sambucus nigra, Spongia tosta, Ipecac, Moschus** at short intervals.

**IF**
- **barking** hoarse cough, starting after a sudden chill
- aggravated by cold drafts
- aggravated at the beginning and end of the night, with perspiration that does not bring relief

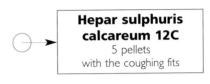

**Hepar sulphuris calcareum 12C**
5 pellets
with the coughing fits

---

## FITFUL COUGH

Spasmodic cough, often similar to cock's crow, occurring in volleys.

**IF**
- violent, **explosive**, spasmodic cough caused by cold air, with
- **choking before the fit**
- **deep red** color of the face
- exhaustion after the fit of coughing, which produces mucus
- aggravation from cold air
- aggravation at night (the patient puts his nose under the blankets to avoid coughing)

**Corallium rubrum 6C**
5 pellets
with the coughing fits

**IF**
- fitful cough **from laryngeal tickling** with
- **discharge of thready mucus**
- aggravation • **before midnight**
  - in the morning on waking
  - in a warm room
- improvement when drinking cold water

**Coccus cacti 6C**
5 pellets
with the coughing fits

**IF**
- short, rapid, hurried, fitful cough, recurring in bouts, preventing the patient from breathing, with sensation of **laryngeal tickling** as from a feather
- aggravation • at night
  - when speaking
  - when drinking
  - when laughing
- improvement • with warmth of the bed
  - **when holding the abdomen to immobilize the ribs**

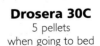

**Drosera 30C**
5 pellets
when going to bed

## LOOSE COUGH

This corresponds to the fully-declared or terminal phase of cough. It is characterized by the formation of mucus, variable in quantity, which may or may not be easy to expel.

**IF** - accumulation of mucus in the bronchi, difficult to expectorate, with
- noisy and impeded breathing, wheezing
- the person is pale, drowsy, dejected, with fluttering of the wings of the nose
- lips are bluish, rings under the eyes
- aggravation • at night
            • when lying
- improvement • with rejection of mucus
            • when sitting

> **Antimonium tartaricum 12C**
> 5 pellets
> 2 to 4 times a day

**IF** - asphyxiating, spasmodic cough, accompanied by **nausea and vomiting**
- **much mucus** in the bronchi
- **clear tongue** despite nausea

> **Ipecac 12C**
> 5 pellets
> 2 to 4 times a day

**IF** - **mucopurulent** loose cough with hypersalivation, **fetid breath**
- **tongue retaining teethmarks,** with yellowish coating at the base
- viscous perspiration which does not bring relief
- aggravation at night

> **Mercurius solubilis 12C**
> 5 pellets
> 2 to 4 times a day

**IF** - loose cough during the day, dry at night
- **loss of sense of taste and smell**
- **improvement with fresh air,**

> **Pulsatilla 12C**
> 5 pellets
> 2 to 4 times a day

- Low dilutions (6C) are used to encourage difficult expectoration.
- High dilutions (12C and higher) are used to diminish bronchial hyper-secretion.

## SPECIALTY

• **CHESTAL®** syrup
Adults and children 12 years and over: 2 teaspoons every 2 hours.
Children 2 to 12 years: 1 teaspoon every 2 hours.
Children under 2: not recommended.

## COUGHS

### DRY COUGH

• **Aconitum napellus 12C**
- sudden high fever
- absence of perspiration

• **Belladonna 12C**
- presence of sweating
- "tumor - rubor - dolor - calor"

• **Bryonia alba 12C**
- aggravation from any movement
- intense thirst
- dryness of mucous membranes

• **Rumex crispus 6C**
- irritation with tickling
- aggravation from cold air

### HOARSE COUGH

• **Hepar sulphuris calcareum 12C**
- barking cough
- aggravation from cold drafts
- sweating does not relieve

• **Spongia tosta 6C**
- dry croupy cough, with wheezing
- noise resembling a saw cutting through pinewood
- dryness, burning of the throat

### FITFUL COUGH

• **Corallium rubrum 6C**
- exhausting, explosive cough
- choking during the fit
- deep red face
- aggravation from cold air (nose under the blankets)

• **Coccus cacti 6C**
- cough due to laryngeal tickling
- production of thready mucus
- aggravation before midnight

• **Drosera 30C**
- cough with laryngeal tickling "as from a feather"
- aggravation when speaking, drinking, laughing, etc.
- improvement when holding the abdomen to immobilize the ribs

### LOOSE COUGH

• **Antimonium tartaricum 12C**
- restricted breathing (from mucus), noisy, wheezing
- pale face
- fluttering of wings of the nose

• **Ipecac 12C**
- asphyxiating cough with nausea and vomiting
- clear tongue
- accumulation of mucus in the bronchi

• **Mercurius solubilis 12C**
- mucopurulent cough
- fetid breath
- tongue retaining teethmarks

• **Pulsatilla 12C**
- loose cough during the day, dry at night
- loss of sense of taste and smell
- improvement with fresh air

# CRAMPS

Cramps are involuntary, painful, and transient contractions of a muscle or a muscular region.

## DETERMINING SYMPTOMS

Suddenness of onset.

Sharp spasmodic pain, becoming paroxysmal (tonic and paralyzing).

**Etiology:**

The causes are varied, but there is often an accumulation of metabolic waste products (lactic acid) in the muscles.

Cramps occur when there is repeated muscular effort bearing either on a muscle or on a neuromuscular axon, which becomes tetanized by asphyxiation.

This is also the case in elderly patients, often caused by a slowing of the circulation (nocturnal cramps).

Certain types of cramp are related to medication, leading to electrolyte imbalance (e.g. potassium depletion due to certain diuretic drugs).

Although they are involuntary, certain types of cramp-like spasmodic muscular contractions are related to psychological factors (emotions, vexations, etc.).

Certain manifestations of a spasmodic and cramping nature are the result of inflammation (pains from hepatic or renal colic, or from spasmodic colitis).

Before any strenuous or sustained effort, athletes (even amateurs!) should pay careful attention to nutritional factors:

1) an ample intake of water;

2) rapidly assimilated simple sugars to support immediate effort;

3) slowly assimilated carbohydrates to accompany prolonged effort;

4) restricted intake of proteins (which lead to the production of nitrogenous waste products).

To prevent muscular fatigue, **Arnica montana**, which is active on the muscles and the capillaries, helps to limit aches and pains and to prolong effort.

The inclusion of **Sarcolacticum acidum 6X** in the **Sporténine** formula counteracts the accumulation of lactic acid in the muscles.

## PRINCIPAL MEDICINES

Before taking any medication, one simple measure to help release the contraction is to apply ice or a refrigerant liquid (sprayed or directly applied on the skin) over the neuromuscular area involved in order to induce vasoconstriction.
Extension of the contracted limb can also release a cramp.

**IF**
- spasmodic cramping pain in a muscle
- aggravated by pressure
- improved when drinking cold water

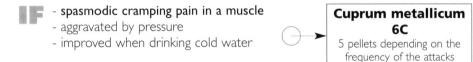

**Cuprum metallicum 6C**
5 pellets depending on the frequency of the attacks

**Cuprum metallicum** is also an excellent medicine for hiccup.

**IF**
- visceral cramping pain, violent but intermittent
- **improved when bending double**
- **improved by strong pressure**
- improved by warmth
- left-sided

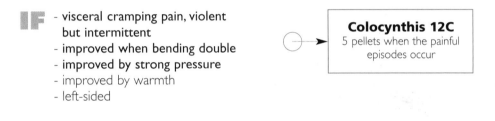

**Colocynthis 12C**
5 pellets when the painful episodes occur

**IF**
- flashing shooting sharp pain, starting and ending rapidly
- improved when bending double (as **Colocynthis**)
- improved by strong local pressure
- improved by warmth
- right-sided

**Magnesia phosphorica 12C**
5 pellets when the spasmodic episodes occur

**Magnesia phosphorica** acts on the neuromuscular axon and on the smooth and striated muscles (writers and musicians' cramps for example).

**IF**
- paroxysmal, cramp-like, acute pain, recurring at regular intervals
- **improved by stretching**

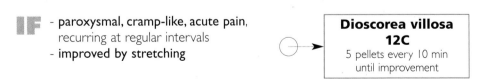

**Dioscorea villosa 12C**
5 pellets every 10 min until improvement

**IF** - cramping menstrual pain, with pain proportional to the menstrual flow

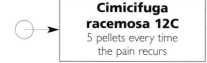

**Cimicifuga racemosa 12C**
5 pellets every time the pain recurs

**Colocynthis** is also a medicine for cramping dysmenorrhea if the patient is improved by bending double.

---

### SPECIALTY

- **LEG CRAMPS CAREKIT** contains Cuprum metallicum 6C, Magnesia phosphorica 6C and Zincum metallicum 6C

---

### CRAMPS

- **Cuprum metallicum 6C**
  - cramping spasmodic pain
  - aggravated by pressure

- **Colocynthis 12C**
  - violent but intermittent visceral pain
  - improvement when bending double
  - left-sided

- **Magnesia phosphorica 12C**
  - the same, but right-sided

- **Dioscorea villosa 12C**
  - paroxysmal acute pain
  - improved by extension

- **Cimicifuga racemosa 12C**
  - menstrual pain

# DELIVERY

Homeopathic medicines can facilitate delivery by acting on two levels:
* physiological,
* psychological (anxiety).


## PRINCIPAL MEDICINES

● *8th month of pregnancy*
- for muscles and capillaries

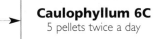
**Arnica montana 12C**
5 pellets a day

- anticipation anxiety before delivery

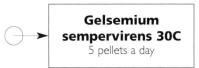
**Gelsemium
sempervirens 30C**
5 pellets a day

--------------------------------------------------------

● *One week before delivery*
- rigidity of the cervix
- spasmodic pains at end
  of pregnancy and postpartum

**Caulophyllum 6C**
5 pellets twice a day

--------------------------------------------------------

● *During delivery*
- strong and irregular delivery pains with
  spasms of the cervix

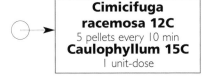
**Cimicifuga
racemosa 12C**
5 pellets every 10 min
**Caulophyllum 15C**
1 unit-dose

--------------------------------------------------------

● *After delivery*
- the following can be continued:

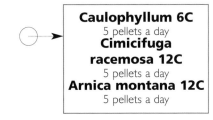
**Caulophyllum 6C**
5 pellets a day
**Cimicifuga
racemosa 12C**
5 pellets a day
**Arnica montana 12C**
5 pellets a day

- to avoid septic complications

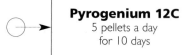

**Pyrogenium 12C**
5 pellets a day
for 10 days

- for exhaustion following profuse
  loss of physiological liquid

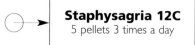

**Cinchona officinalis
12C**
5 pellets a day

- in case of cesarean section
  or episiotomy

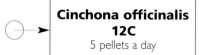

**Staphysagria 12C**
5 pellets 3 times a day

- in cases of postpartum depression

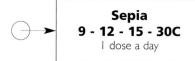

**Sepia
9 - 12 - 15 - 30C**
1 dose a day

## DELIVERY: before - during - after

- **Gelsemium sempervirens 30C**
  - anticipation anxiety

- **Arnica montana 12C**
  - contusion, ecchymosis

- **Caulophyllum 6C**
  - rigidity or spasm of the cervix

- **Cimicifuga racemosa 12C**
  - pains

- **Pyrogenium 12C**
  - infection

- **Cinchona officinalis 12C**
  - fatigue

- **Staphysagria 12C**
  - clean cuts

- **Sepia 9 - 12 - 15 - 30C**
  - postpartum depression

# DENTAL PROBLEMS

## PRINCIPAL MEDICINES

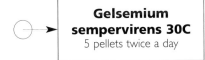 - **anxiety**, fear of going to the dentist, postponement of appointments

→ **Gelsemium sempervirens 30C**
5 pellets twice a day

This medicine often helps patients to undergo dental treatment without difficulties.

**IF** - **beginning of abscess**, swollen, painful, red mucosa

→ **Belladonna 6C**
5 pellets 4 times a day

**IF** - risk of infection

→ **Pyrogenium 12C**
5 pellets twice a day

**IF** - **tooth extraction**

### • 3 days before the intervention

- for traumatism

→ **Arnica montana 12C**
5 pellets twice a day

- for anxiety

→ **Gelsemium sempervirens 30C**
5 pellets twice a day

- for hemorrhaging

→ **Phosphorus 30C**
5 pellets twice a day

### • after the intervention

- continue

→ **Arnica montana 12C**
5 pellets 3 times a day

- to prevent alveolitis, add

→ **Hypericum perforatum 30C**
5 pellets 3 times a day

- in case of hyperesthesia to pain

→ **Chamomilla 30C**
5 pellets 3 times a day

**IF** - **inflammation of the oral mucosa**, with progressive receding of gums (periodontitis)

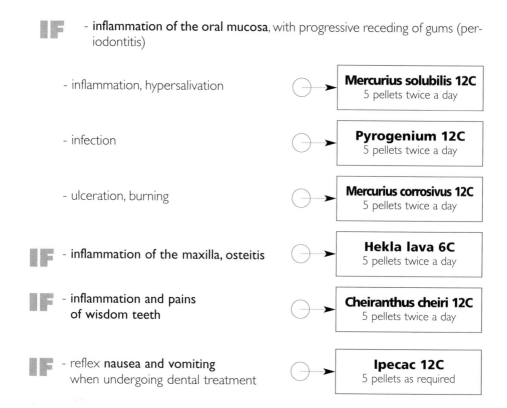

- inflammation, hypersalivation → **Mercurius solubilis 12C**
  5 pellets twice a day

- infection → **Pyrogenium 12C**
  5 pellets twice a day

- ulceration, burning → **Mercurius corrosivus 12C**
  5 pellets twice a day

**IF** - **inflammation of the maxilla, osteitis** → **Hekla lava 6C**
  5 pellets twice a day

**IF** - **inflammation and pains of wisdom teeth** → **Cheiranthus cheiri 12C**
  5 pellets twice a day

**IF** - reflex **nausea and vomiting** when undergoing dental treatment → **Ipecac 12C**
  5 pellets as required

---

## TEETHING IN CHILDREN

### DETERMINING SYMPTOMS

Inflammation of the mucous membranes, fever, behavioral disorders due to the pain.

## PRINCIPAL MEDICINES

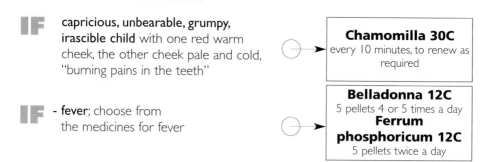

**IF** capricious, unbearable, grumpy, irascible child with one red warm cheek, the other cheek pale and cold, "burning pains in the teeth" → **Chamomilla 30C**
every 10 minutes, to renew as required

**IF** - **fever**; choose from the medicines for fever → **Belladonna 12C**
5 pellets 4 or 5 times a day
**Ferrum phosphoricum 12C**
5 pellets twice a day

- digestive disorders with diarrhea
  (due to teething)

> **Rheum officinale 12C**
> **Podophyllum 12C**
> 5 pellets after every bowel
> movement

## SPECIALTY

- **CAMILIA®**: Children 4 months of age and older: I single dose every 15 minutes for 3 doses.

## DENTAL PROBLEMS

- **Gelsemium sempervirens 30C**
  - anxiety, fear of the idea of going to the dentist

- **Belladonna 6C**
  - beginning of abscess
  - red, painful, swollen mucosa

- **Pyrogenium 12C**
  - to prevent infection

### DENTAL EXTRACTION

**3 DAYS BEFORE INTERVENTION**

- **Arnica montana 12C**
  - for traumatism

- **Gelsemium sempervirens 30C**
  - for anxiety

- **Phosphorus 30C**
  - for hemorrhaging

**AFTER INTERVENTION**

- **Arnica montana 12C and Hypericum perforatum 30C**
  - to prevent risks of alveolitis

- **Chamomilla 30C**
  - in case of hyperesthesia to pain

**INFLAMMATION**

- **Mercurius solubilis 12C**
  - inflammation, hypersalivation

- **Pyrogenium 12C**
  - infection

- **Mercurius corrosivus 12C**
  - ulceration, burning

- **Hekla lava 6C**
  - inflammation of maxilla, osteitis

- **Cheiranthus cheiri 12C**
  - inflammation and pains of wisdom teeth

- **Ipecac 12C**
  - nausea, vomiting

### TEETHING IN CHILDREN

- **Chamomilla 30C**
  - capricious, unbearable, grumpy, irascible child
  - one warm red cheek, the other pale and cold
  - "burning pains in teeth"

- **Belladonna 12C or Ferrum phosphoricum 12C**
  - when there is fever

- **Rheum officinale 12C Podophyllum 12C**
  - when accompanied by digestive disorders with diarrhea

# DERMATOSIS

The generic name of dermatosis can be applied to all skin diseases. These conditions have the advantage of being readily visible, so the choice of the medicine is easier.
Dermatoses range from simple dermatitis (inflammatory reaction of the skin, such as insect bites or stings) to much deeper manifestations (chronic eczema) or severe disorders (skin cancer).

## DETERMINING SYMPTOMS

- Aspect of the lesions (papules, vesicles, phlyctenae, fissures, scales, consistency and smell of any discharge, scabs, etc.)
- Etiology when direct.
- Modalities of improvement or aggravation of the lesions from scratching, warmth, cold, water, etc.
- Chronic dermatosis related to constitutional factors must be treated by the physician.

In some specific cases, advice from the pharmacist may be sufficient, especially when the etiology is known.

## PRINCIPAL MEDICINES

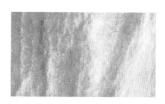

### ERYTHEMATOUS AND/OR EDEMATOUS DERMATOSIS

**IF**
- **burning edema**, stinging, pruritic, pinkish-red
- improvement by applying cold water
  insect bites or stings, sunburns, first-degree burns, urticaria

→ **Apis mellifica 12C**
5 pellets 4 or 5 times a day

**IF**
- **burning edema**, stinging, pruritic
- aggravation by applying cold water
  urticaria of allergic, alimentary, toxic, or contact origin

→ **Urtica urens 6C**
5 pellets 4 or 5 times a day

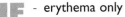 - **pruriginous erythema** of the skin related to cold
- sensation of stinging, burning, itching, and tingling
  chilblains

→ **Agaricus muscarius 6C**
5 pellets 4 or 5 times a day

**IF** - **erythema only**
- "tumor – rubor – dolor - calor" (tumefaction, redness, pain, heat)
  first-degree burns with **Apis mellifica**

→ **Belladonna 6C**
5 pellets 4 or 5 times a day

---

## VESICULAR DERMATOSIS

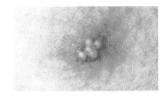

---

**IF** - **small-size vesicles filled with a transparent lemon-yellow liquid**, on a red skin
- improvement by **applying very hot water**
- **no improvement with scratching**
  herpes, chickenpox, herpes zoster

→ **Rhus toxicodendron 12C**
5 pellets 3 or 4 times a day

**IF** - vesicular eruption with an **opalescent** liquid
- **scabs on the lesions**, with underlying yellowish serous fluid
  herpes, herpes zoster

→ **Mezereum 12C**
5 pellets 3 or 4 times a day

**IF** - vesicles or pustules (like impetigo) situated **around the mouth**

→ **Antimonium crudum 12C**
5 pellets 3 or 4 times a day

**IF** - numerous vesicles grouped together with **itching** of the hands and fingers
  palmar and digital dyshidrosis

→ **Anagallis arvensis 12C**
5 pellets 3 or 4 times a day

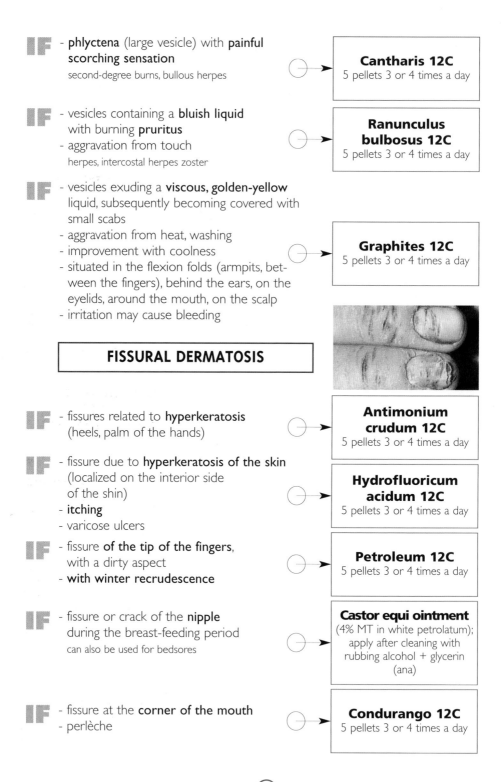

**IF** - phlyctena (large vesicle) with **painful scorching sensation**
second-degree burns, bullous herpes

**Cantharis 12C**
5 pellets 3 or 4 times a day

**IF** - vesicles containing a **bluish liquid** with burning **pruritus**
- aggravation from touch
herpes, intercostal herpes zoster

**Ranunculus bulbosus 12C**
5 pellets 3 or 4 times a day

**IF** - vesicles exuding a **viscous, golden-yellow** liquid, subsequently becoming covered with small scabs
- aggravation from heat, washing
- improvement with coolness
- situated in the flexion folds (armpits, between the fingers), behind the ears, on the eyelids, around the mouth, on the scalp
- irritation may cause bleeding

**Graphites 12C**
5 pellets 3 or 4 times a day

## FISSURAL DERMATOSIS

**IF** - fissures related to **hyperkeratosis** (heels, palm of the hands)

**Antimonium crudum 12C**
5 pellets 3 or 4 times a day

**IF** - fissure due to **hyperkeratosis of the skin** (localized on the interior side of the shin)
- **itching**
- varicose ulcers

**Hydrofluoricum acidum 12C**
5 pellets 3 or 4 times a day

**IF** - fissure **of the tip of the fingers**, with a dirty aspect
- **with winter recrudescence**

**Petroleum 12C**
5 pellets 3 or 4 times a day

**IF** - fissure or crack of the **nipple** during the breast-feeding period
can also be used for bedsores

**Castor equi ointment**
(4% MT in white petrolatum); apply after cleaning with rubbing alcohol + glycerin (ana)

**IF** - fissure at the **corner of the mouth**
- perlèche

**Condurango 12C**
5 pellets 3 or 4 times a day

**IF** - fissure with **clear edges, bleeding**
readily if touched, on **yellow** and indurated integument
- situated on the skin or
at the **mucocutaneous junction**
- aggravation from cold, touch
- improvement with warmth

> **Nitricum acidum**
> **12C**
> 5 pellets 3 or 4 times a day

**IF** - slit in the middle of the lower lip

> **Natrum muriaticum**
> **12C**
> 5 pellets 3 or 4 times a day

## SQUAMOUS DERMATOSIS

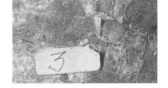

**IF** - **fine, purpuric, dry** scales
(desquamation resembles bran)
- dandruffs
- eczema

> **Arsenicum album**
> **12C**
> 5 pellets 3 or 4 times a day

**IF** - fine **transparent** scales, tearing off
**in large strips**
- with **red underlying dermis**
**which shines as if wet**
- palmar or plantar dyshidrosis

> **Natrum sulphuricum**
> **12C**
> 5 pellets 3 or 4 times a day

## CIRCINATE DERMATOSIS

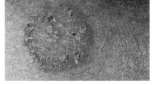

**IF** - dermatosis **in a circular shape**, limited
at the outside by a reddish zone, more
or less embossed, intact in the center
- mycosis
- circinate herpes

> **Berberis vulgaris 6C**
> 5 pellets 3 or 4 times a day

- **ERYTHEMA**: CALENDULA CREAM, apply a thin layer 2 or 3 times a day
- **BURNS, CRACKED SKIN**: CALENDULA OINTMENT, apply a thin layer 2 or 3 times a day

## DERMATOSIS

### ERYTHEMA

- **Apis mellifica 12C**
  - insect bites or stings
  - sunburns
  - urticaria
  - improvement by applying cold water

- **Urtica urens 6C**
  - the same, but aggravation by applying cold water

- **Agaricus muscarius 6C**
  - pruriginous erythema related to cold
  - chilblains

- **Belladonna 6C**
  - "tumor - rubor - dolor - calor"

### VESICULAR ERUPTION

- **Rhus toxicodendron 12C**
  - small-size vesicles
  - transparent liquid
  - herpes, herpes zoster, chickenpox

- **Mezereum 12C**
  - vesicles with a cloudy liquid and yellowish serous fluid
  - herpes, herpes zoster, chickenpox

- **Antimonium crudum 12C**
  - pustules resembling impetigo around the mouth

- **Anagallis arvensis 12C**
  - vesicles with itching of the hands and fingers

- **Cantharis 12C**
  - large vesicles
  - scorching pain
  - second-degree burns
  - bullous herpes

- **Ranunculus bulbosus 12C**
  - vesicles containing a bluish liquid
  - pruritus
  - aggravation from touch
  - intercostal herpes zoster
  - herpes

- **Graphites 12C**
  - vesicles exuding a viscous, golden-yellow liquid
  - often in the folds
  - improvement with coolness

### FISSURES

- **Antimonium crudum 12C**
  - hyperkeratosis (heels)

- **Hydrofluoricum acidum 12C**
  - with itching
  - varicose ulcers

- **Petroleum 12C**
  - tip of the fingers
  - dirty aspect
  - often related to cold

- **Castor equi ointment**
  - fissure or crack of the nipple ( breast-feeding)
  - bedsores

- **Condurango 12C**
  - corner of the mouth

- **Nitricum acidum 12C**
  - fissure with clear edges, bleeding readily

- **Natrum muriaticum 12C**
  - slit in the middle of the lower lip

### SQUAMOUS ERUPTION

- **Arsenicum album 12C**
  - fine, purpuric, dry scales (resembling bran)
  - dandruff
  - eczema

- **Natrum sulphuricum 12C**
  - fine, transparent scales, in large strips
  - shiny red underlying dermis
  - palmar or plantar dyshidrosis

## ERYTHEMATOUS AND/OR EDEMATOUS DERMATOSIS

- **Apis mellifica 12C**
  - burning, stinging, pruritic edema
  - improvement with cold applications

- **Urtica urens 6C**
  - burning, stinging, pruritic edema
  - aggravation from cold applications

- **Agaricus muscarius 6C**
  - pruritus related to cold
  - chilblains
  - stings, burns, itching, tingling

- **Belladonna 6C**
  - pain, heat, tumefaction

## VESICULAR DERMATOSIS

- **Rhus toxicodendron 12C**
  - small vesicles
  - light lemon-yellow liquid
  - improvement by applying very hot water
  - no improvement with scratching

- **Mezereum 12C**
  - vesicles with a cloudy liquid
  - scabs and underlying serous fluid

- **Antimonium crudum 12C**
  - vesicles around the mouth
  - yellow serous fluid and scabs

- **Anagallis arvensis12C**
  - small vesicles, numerous, grouped together, with itching of the hands and fingers

- **Ranunculus bulbosus 12C**
  - vesicles with a hematic liquid, pruritic, burning
  - aggravation from touch

- **Graphites 12C**
  - vesicles with a honey-yellow liquid, small scabs
  - aggravation from heat, washing
  - improvement with coolness

- **Cantharis 12C**
  - burning phlyctenae and pain

## FISSURAL DERMATOSIS

- **Antimonium crudum 12C**
  - fissures due to hyperkeratosis
  - heels, palms of the hands

- **Hydrofluoricum acidum 12C**
  - fissures with hyperkeratosis (interior side of shin), itching
  - varicose ulcers

- **Petroleum 12C**
  - fissures of the tip of the fingers with winter recrudescence

- **Castor equi ointment**
  - cracked nipple after breast-feeding
  - bedsores

- **Condurango 12C**
  - fissure at the corner of the mouth
  - perlèche

- **Nitricum acidum 12C**
  - distinct fissure on the skin or at the mucocutaneous junction, clear edges
  - bleeding from touch
  - yellow integument

- **Natrum muriaticum 12C**
  - fissure of the lower lip

## SQUAMOUS DERMATOSIS

- **Arsenicum album 12C**
  - small scales, like bran

- **Natrum sulphuricum 12C**
  - large scales in transparent strips
  - shiny red underlying skin, as if wet

## CIRCINATE DERMATOSIS

- **Berberis vulgaris 6C**
  - dermatosis with a circular shape
  - peripheral red area
  - intact central area

# DIARRHEA

Diarrhea is characterized by frequent and liquid stools.

The repeated evacuation of normal stools does not constitute diarrhea.

**Diarrhea is not a disease, but a symptom for which the cause or causes must be sought.**

Pharmacists or nurses can only intervene on an ad hoc basis, in cases of acute diarrhea with clear causes.

The treatment of chronic diarrhea should be left to a qualified physician.

Diarrhea can be more or less serious, depending on the age and the general condition of the patient.

Infant diarrhea, which leads rapidly to dehydration, must be halted promptly and receive proper medical attention.

## DETERMINING SYMPTOMS

**Acute diarrhea from a known cause, such as:**
- food or drink taken; or
- circumstances interrupting or blocking the digestion, for example taking cold drinks during digestion or heatstroke.

Diarrhea can also be related to the misuse of laxatives or of certain medicines (such as colchicine), leading to frothy, acidic stools, due to a phenomenon of osmosis.

Acute diarrhea is often of bacterial or viral origin; it may also be a symptom of parasitic infestation (amebiasis).

The pharmacist must be careful to establish the benign nature of the diarrhea, and can only give treatment advice if the cause is clear.

## PRINCIPAL MEDICINES

 - exhausting painless diarrhea
  with foul-smelling gas
- **bloating of the whole abdomen**
- caused by the ingestion of milk, alcohol,
  acidic food or drinks

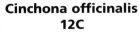

**Cinchona officinalis
12C**
5 pellets after each bowel
movement

**Cinchona officinalis** is indicated in all cases of loss of organic fluid leading to weakness, making it useful in all types of diarrhea.

**IF** - **brownish** diarrhea (like prune juice), **burning, foul-smelling**, related to food poisoning (spoiled meat, pâté, mussels, sea food, fruit)

> **Arsenicum album 12C**
> 5 pellets after each bowel movement

**IF** - **spurting** diarrhea, frequent, **exhausting**, with cold sweats, cramping abdominal pains

> **Veratrum album 12C**
> 5 pellets after each bowel movement

It is advisable for travelers, especially to hot countries, to have **Arsenicum album** and **Veratrum album** on hand, to be taken as first-line therapy.

**IF** - diarrhea with stools of **variable consistency** related to the ingestion of **cakes, ice-creams**

> **Pulsatilla 12C**
> 5 pellets after each bowel movement

**IF** - **half-solid, half-liquid diarrhea**, related to overeating, acidic foods, or after a cold bath interrupting the digestion

> **Antimonium crudum 12C**
> 5 pellets after each bowel movement

**IF** - exhausting watery diarrhea, with cramping pain, very often in the morning **after excessive consumption of fresh fruit** or food poisoning (turista)
- bloating of the right iliac fossa
- nausea

> **Podophyllum 12C**
> 5 pellets after each bowel movement

**IF** - **frothy, fermented stools, green like grass, nausea**
- hypersalivation

> **Ipecac 12C**
> 5 pellets after each bowel movement

**IF** - frothy green diarrhea (**like frog spawn**), irritant, caused by milk (in children who do not tolerate milk)

> **Magnesia carbonica 12C**
> 5 pellets after each bowel movement

**IF** - diarrhea **related to teething** or after excessive consumption of unripe fruit
- sour smell
- brown and clay-like stools

> **Rheum officinale 12C**
> 5 pellets after each bowel movement

- diarrhea **with mucus**
- urgent, spurting
- aggravated by food, drink
- **much rumbling and gas**

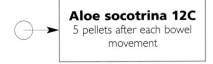

**Aloe socotrina 12C**
5 pellets after each bowel movement

All these homeopathic medicines can be given as first-line therapy. If normalization does not follow within the next few hours, refer to the physician.

---

## DIARRHEA

● **Cinchona officinalis 12C**
- painless
- exhausting
- the whole abdomen is bloated

● **Arsenicum album 12C**
- burning
- foul-smelling
- following food poisoning

● **Veratrum album 12C**
- ejected in spurts
- exhausting
- cramping pains in the abdomen

● **Pulsatilla 12C**
- variable consistency
  (from ice-creams, cakes)

● **Antimonium crudum 12C**
- half-solid, half-liquid
- following overeating
- after a cold bath interrupting the
  digestion

● **Podophyllum 12C**
- watery
- exhausting
- cramping pains

● **Ipecac 12C**
- green, fermented, frothy (like grass)
- nausea

● **Magnesia carbonica 12C**
- green, frothy (frog spawn)
- caused by milk
  (children intolerant to milk)

● **Rheum officinale 12C**
- brown, clay-like
- due to excessive consumption
  of unripe fruit
- teething

● **Aloe socotrina 12C**
- with mucus
- urgent, spurting
- much rumbling and gas

# DIGESTIVE DISORDERS

Disorders of the digestive functions may be:

## 1) Sudden and passing in nature
(indigestion, occasional diarrhea)

These disorders are usually caused by exogenous factors:
- overeating or drinking;
- intolerance to certain foods;
- intoxication;
- blockage of digestion by atmospheric conditions (cold or sunshine), or by emotional factors and vexations.

## 2) Repetitive in nature
(related to the individual constitution or to poor dietary habits)

The repetition of functional disorders can lead to lesional conditions, stomach ulcers, colitis, hepatic and biliary colic, diabetes, cancer.

 **The advisory role of pharmacists should be limited to transitory disorders.**

Any recurring condition will require a thorough exploration of the digestive functions.
The health care professional  can provide an important service by seeking to pinpoint dietary errors, and by giving appropriate dietary advice.

# INDIGESTION

Sudden and transitory blocking of digestive functions.

## DETERMINING SYMPTOMS

- general malaise,
- cold perspiration,
- nausea,
- sometimes vomiting, hiccup, followed by colic, diarrhea.

**Etiology:**
- food, or
- exogenous factors: cold, heat, exposure to the sun, bath, vexation, etc.; or
- intolerance of certain foods.

## PRINCIPAL MEDICINES

**IF**
- **tongue white all over** (as after drinking milk)
- belching with the taste of ingested foods
- half-solid, half-liquid diarrhea
- aggravation from excessive eating
  from cold bath
  from heat (sun, heat stroke)

**Antimonium crudum 12C**
5 pellets 2 or 3 times a day

This medicine corresponds to big eaters, more interested in quantity than in quality.

**IF**
- **tongue white at the back**
- postprandial drowsiness
- sensation of a stone in the stomach
- nausea relieved by vomiting
- aggravation from alcohol
  from tobacco
  from spices
- belching

**Nux vomica 12C**
5 pellets 2 or 3 times a day

This medicine corresponds to individuals who prefer quality to quantity when eating; they are irritable because of their hectic lifestyle.

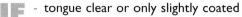

**IF**
- **tongue clear or only slightly coated**
- nausea, vomiting (which does not relieve the nausea)
- hypersalivation
- diarrhea after ingestion of unripe fruit
- disgust for all foods

○ ➤ | **Ipecac 12C**
5 pellets 2 or 3 times a day |

The toxicology includes vomiting.

**IF**
- digestive function is blocked following **vexation**

○ ➤ | **Ignatia amara 12C**
5 pellets 2 or 3 times a day |

**IF**
- digestive function is blocked following **anger**, with **spasms**

○ ➤ | **Colocynthis 12C**
5 pellets 2 or 3 times a day |

## FOOD INTOLERANCE

Indigestion is sometimes related to an individual's sensitivity to a given food, even in small quantities; it may also by caused by excessive consumption.

## PRINCIPAL MEDICINES

**IF**
- intolerance to **wine, spirits**, stimulants

○ ➤ | **Nux vomica 12C**
5 pellets twice a day |

**IF**
- intolerance to **vinegary** foods

○ ➤ | **Antimonium crudum 12C**
5 pellets twice a day |

**IF**
- intolerance to **fruits**

○ ➤ | **Arsenicum album 12C**
5 pellets twice a day |

**IF**
- intolerance to **oysters**, garlic, onions

○ ➤ | **Lycopodium 12C**
5 pellets twice a day |

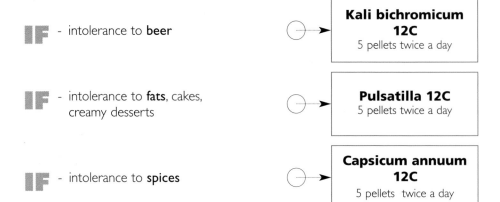

**IF** - intolerance to **beer**

> **Kali bichromicum 12C**
> 5 pellets twice a day

**IF** - intolerance to **fats**, cakes, creamy desserts

> **Pulsatilla 12C**
> 5 pellets twice a day

**IF** - intolerance to **spices**

> **Capsicum annuum 12C**
> 5 pellets twice a day

---

## FOOD POISONING

Food poisoning is most often caused by the ingestion of spoiled food (bacterial pollution) or chemically contaminated food (products used for treating fruit and vegetables).

It can also be caused by naturally toxic foods such as certain mushrooms.

The pharmacist or the nurse must therefore seek to ascertain the cause; if this cannot be determined, **refer to the physician.**

### PRINCIPAL MEDICINES

**IF** - food toxic infection related to meat, spoiled pâté, fish, mussels, seafood
- blackish **foul-smelling burning** diarrhea
- great fatigue

> **Arsenicum album 12C**
> 5 pellets after each bowel movement

**IF** - **spurting** choleriform diarrhea
- **cold sweating**
- dehydration
- **abdominal cramping pains**

> **Veratrum album 12C**
> 5 pellets after each bowel movement twice a day

## RECURRENT DIGESTIVE DISORDERS

 The repetition of digestive disorders, with or without pain, can be an important sign of an underlying grave condition. The patient must be encouraged to consult a doctor if necessary.

The questioning will be focused principally on:
- repeated self-medication without lasting disappearance of the disorders;
- the length of time the disorders have been present;
- the location of pain, if present (e.g. pains in the epigastric region often reflect a disorder of the gall bladder);
- the modalities of appearance and disappearance of the pain or the disorders (e.g. stomach ulcer calmed by eating);
- accompanying general signs suggesting the possibility of a more serious condition (e.g. appendicitis if there is pain in the right iliac fossa or more rarely on the left, coated tongue, urge to vomit);
- unspectacular symptoms, as constant dull pain, stubborn constipation, alternating diarrhea and constipation, black stools resulting from hemorrhaging high up in the digestive tract, red stools from low hemorrhaging or from hemorrhoids, or digestive discomfort after meals with nausea, headaches during the biliary digestive phase suggesting possible spasmodic disorders of Oddi's sphincter, or even gallstones.

Taking note of all these symptoms will help the pharmacist to encourage the person to consult a physician rather than resorting to self-medication.

## MINOR DIGESTIVE DISORDERS

Certain dyspeptic disorders can be considered as minor, when they occur only occasionally, and are directly linked to food intake or to external circumstances affecting digestion.

### 1) Aerophagia
This term, which is not strictly appropriate, designates the accumulation of air throughout the digestive tract (*aero* = air, *phagein* = to eat).
This presence of air is the result of either:
- swallowing air while chewing;
- swallowing air outside meals through a reflex act;
- formation of gas by fermentation.

According to the location of the air, the condition can be described as
- gastric bloating, when the upper parts are affected;
- colonic bloating, when the lower parts are affected.

### 2) Gastric acidity

## PRINCIPAL MEDICINES

### Aerophagia

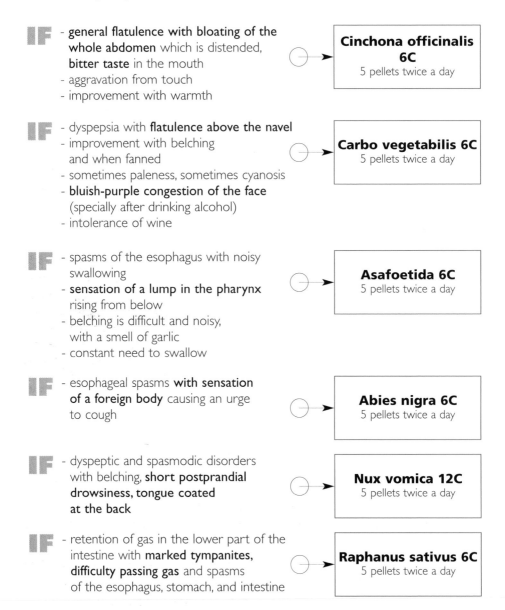

**IF**
- general flatulence with bloating of the whole abdomen which is distended, **bitter taste** in the mouth
- aggravation from touch
- improvement with warmth

**Cinchona officinalis 6C**
5 pellets twice a day

**IF**
- dyspepsia with **flatulence above the navel**
- improvement with belching and when fanned
- sometimes paleness, sometimes cyanosis
- **bluish-purple congestion of the face** (specially after drinking alcohol)
- intolerance of wine

**Carbo vegetabilis 6C**
5 pellets twice a day

**IF**
- spasms of the esophagus with noisy swallowing
- **sensation of a lump in the pharynx** rising from below
- belching is difficult and noisy, with a smell of garlic
- constant need to swallow

**Asafoetida 6C**
5 pellets twice a day

**IF**
- esophageal spasms **with sensation of a foreign body** causing an urge to cough

**Abies nigra 6C**
5 pellets twice a day

**IF**
- dyspeptic and spasmodic disorders with belching, **short postprandial drowsiness, tongue coated at the back**

**Nux vomica 12C**
5 pellets twice a day

**IF**
- retention of gas in the lower part of the intestine with **marked tympanites, difficulty passing gas** and spasms of the esophagus, stomach, and intestine

**Raphanus sativus 6C**
5 pellets twice a day

**Raphanus sativus** accelerates the expulsion of gas after surgical interventions, in combination with **Cinchona officinalis**.

**IF**
- intestinal flatulence
- burning of the esophagus with belching and reflux of acidic and burning liquid
- migraine
- **long postprandial drowsiness**
- aggravation around 5 p.m.

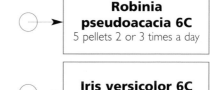

| **Lycopodium 12C** |
| :---: |
| 5 pellets a day |

## Gastric acidity

**IF**
- **acidic reflux**, specially at night
- hyperchlorhydria

| **Robinia pseudoacacia 6C** |
| :---: |
| 5 pellets 2 or 3 times a day |

**IF**
- **burning** of the entire digestive tract
- belching, nausea, vomiting
- profuse salivation

| **Iris versicolor 6C** |
| :---: |
| 5 pellets 2 or 3 times a day |

## SPECIALTIES

- **GASALIA®**: Adults and children 6 years and over, dissolve 2 tablets in the mouth at the onset of symptoms. Repeat if needed every 15 minutes for 3 more doses. Then if necessary take 2 tablets 15 minutes before meal.
- **ACIDIL®**: Adults and children 6 years and over, dissolve 2 tablets in the mouth at the onset of symptoms. Repeat if needed every 15 minutes for 3 more doses. Then if necessary take 2 tablets 15 minutes before meal.
- **AVENOC®** tablets, ointment or suppositories for minor symptoms of hemorrhoids such as soreness, itching and burning.

---

## IRRITABLE BOWEL SYNDROME

Spasmodic colitis is essentially a problem for the physician.

The pharmacist is often consulted for intestinal spasms, related to diet.

This condition is favored by summer foods, acidic foods, foods preserved in brine (green olives), vinegar, spices, spicy sausages, by raw acidic fruits (cherries, raspberries, blackcurrants, redcurrants, as well as tomatoes and melons), and by acidic drinks (rosé wine, champagne, and carbonated drinks containing citric acid).

The health care professional should set out some basic dietary principles.

The daily use of laxatives is a factor which can lead to colitis.

Self-medication with spasmolytic drugs, without taking into account of the dangers of an inappropriate diet, is harmful (the spasm should be considered as a defensive reaction to inflammation).

If all the dietary shortcomings cannot be pinpointed, a "plastering" of the digestive tract with conventional protective or absorbent preparations will help protect against the effects of dietary deviations.


## PRINCIPAL MEDICINES

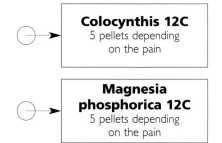

**IF** - spasmodic disorders with violent **cramping pains, generally left-sided, relieved when bending double**

→ **Colocynthis 12C**
5 pellets depending on the pain

**IF** - spasmodic disorders with violent **cramping pains, generally right-sided, relieved when bending double**

→ **Magnesia phosphorica 12C**
5 pellets depending on the pain


### DIGESTIVE DISORDERS

#### OCCASIONAL DIGESTIVE DISORDERS

**INDIGESTION**

• **Antimonium crudum 12C**
- white tongue (milk)
- belching with the taste of food ingested
- often problems with the quantity ingested

• **Nux vomica 12C**
- tongue white at the back
- postprandial drowsiness

• **Ipecac 12C**
- clear tongue
- nausea, vomiting

• **Ignatia amara 12C**
- blocking of digestion following vexation

• **Colocynthis 12C**
- blocking of digestion following anger

**FOOD INTOLERANCE**

• **Nux vomica 12C**
- wine, spirits, stimulants

• **Antimonium crudum 12C**
- vinegary foods

• **Arsenicum album 12C**
- fruit

• **Lycopodium 12C**
- oysters, garlic, onion

- **Kali bichromicum 12C**
  - beer

- **Pulsatilla 12C**
  - fats, cakes, creamy desserts

- **Capsicum annuum 12C**
  - spices

### FOOD POISONING

- **Arsenicum album 12C**
  - Foul-smelling, burning diarrhea

- **Veratrum album 12C**
  - Spurting diarrhea, abdominal pains, cold sweats

## RECURRENT DIGESTIVE DISORDERS

### AEROPHAGIA

- **Cinchona officinalis 6C**
  - flatulence
  - bloating of the entire abdomen

- **Carbo vegetabilis 6C**
  - flatulence above the navel
  - improvement with belching

- **Asafoetida 6C**
  - spasms of the esophagus
  - belching with a garlicky smell

- **Abies nigra 6C**
  - spasms of the esophagus
  - sensation of foreign body, cough

- **Nux vomica 12C**
  - coated tongue at the back
  - postprandial drowsiness
  - dyspepsia

### ACCUMULATION OF GAS IN THE COLON

- **Raphanus sativus 6C**
  - gas retained in the lower part of the intestine (useful after surgery)

- **Lycopodium 12C**
  - intestinal flatulence
  - burning + acidic reflux
  - migraine

### GASTRIC ACIDITY

- **Robinia pseudoacacia 6C**
  - acidic reflux, specially at night

- **Iris versicolor 6C**
  - burning, nausea

### IRRITABLE BOWEL SYNDROME

- **Colocynthis 12C**
  - cramping spasmodic pains
  - improvement when bending forward
  - pain on the left

- **Magnesia phosphorica 12C**
  - spasmodic disorders
  - cramping pains
  - pain on the right
  - improvement when bending double

# EPISTAXIS (NOSEBLEED)

Epistaxis, or nosebleed, is a hemorrhage of the mucous membranes of the nasal passages.

## DETERMINING SYMPTOMS

The etiology of the nasal hemorrhage should be sought.
The cause can be local:
- blow,
- traumatism,
- cysts inside the nostrils;
or general:
- sunstroke,
- high blood pressure,
- after-effects of infectious diseases.

Some hemorrhages with a general cause represent a physiological means of regulation and should therefore be respected.

To stop the hemorrhage when necessary, the following can be done:
- local pressure on the wing of the nose;
- vasoconstriction from cold (ice cubes);
- implementation of a wick impregnated with an anti-hemorrhagic substance (alginate or hydrogen peroxide).

## PRINCIPAL MEDICINES

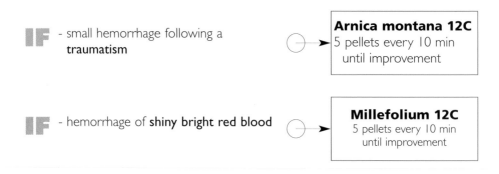

**IF** - small hemorrhage following a **traumatism** → **Arnica montana 12C** 5 pellets every 10 min until improvement

**IF** - hemorrhage of **shiny bright red blood** → **Millefolium 12C** 5 pellets every 10 min until improvement

It is possible to alternate **Arnica montana** and **Millefolium**, 5 pellets every 10 minutes.

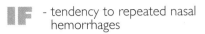 - tendency to repeated nasal hemorrhages

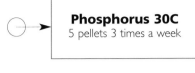

**Phosphorus 30C**
5 pellets 3 times a week

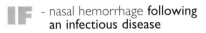 - nasal hemorrhage **following an infectious disease**

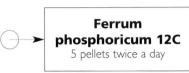

**Ferrum phosphoricum 12C**
5 pellets twice a day

In all cases, **Cinchona officinalis** is the medicine for loss of physiological fluid.

---

## EPISTAXIS

- **Arnica montana 12C**
  - hemorrhage following a traumatism

- **Millefolium 12C**
  - hemorrhage of shiny bright red blood

- **Ferrum phosphoricum 12C**
  - hemorrhage due to an infectious disease

- **Phosphorus 30C**
  - tendency to repeated nasal hemorrhages

### IN ALL CASES

- **Cinchona officinalis 12C**
  - to fight against anemia and fatigue following a loss of physiological or pathological liquid

# FELON

Felon is an inflammation of the fingertip (sometimes toe), following a scratch, a sting or a piercing wound; it evolves towards infection.
There are several stages of felon from superficial circumscribed whitlow to deep felon involving the synovial sheaths of the bones and joints of the fingers or toes.

## DETERMINING SYMPTOMS

These depend on a visual evaluation, and essentially on the evolution which can be predicted, but also on an appreciation of the general condition.

 The pharmacist is only competent to deal with cases of superficial felon, which do not require any surgical intervention.

## LOCAL TREATMENT

Repeated, warm, local baths, or damp dressings with **Calendula MT.**

## PRINCIPAL MEDICINES

**IF**
- inflammation with redness and **throbbing pains**
- "tumor - rubor - dolor - calor"

**Belladonna 12C**
5 pellets 3 or 4 times a day

**IF**
- red shiny finger, with **stinging pains** as from red-hot needles
- hypersensitivity to touch
- aggravation of the pain from heat
- **improvement with cold**

**Apis mellifica 12C**
5 pellets 3 or 4 times a day

**IF**
- inflammation following **stings or bites, or from puncture of the skin without bleeding**

**Ledum palustre 6C**
5 pellets 3 or 4 times a day

- In all cases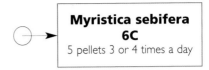

**Myristica sebifera 6C**
5 pellets 3 or 4 times a day

is the principal medicine for felons, as it facilitates the opening of the abscess and the drainage of pus.

- helps with draining of the discharge after excision

**Calcarea sulphurica 6C**
5 pellets 3 or 4 times a day

- stops the infection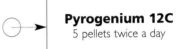

**Pyrogenium 12C**
5 pellets twice a day

---

## FELON

### LOCALLY

- **Calendula MT**
  - repeated warm baths, or damp dressings

- **Belladonna 12C**
  - inflammation with redness
  - throbbing pains
  - "tumor - rubor - dolor - calor"
  - improvement with warm applications
  - aggravation from cold

- **Apis mellifica 12C**
  - shiny red finger
  - stinging pains as from red-hot needles
  - improvement with cold
  - aggravation from warm applications

- **Ledum palustre 6C**
  - inflammation following stings or bites, or puncture of the skin without bleeding

### IN ALL CASES

- **Myristica sebifera 6C**
  - facilitates opening of the felon and drainage of pus

### AFTER EXCISION

- **Calcarea sulphurica 6C**
  - helps to drain the discharge

- **Pyrogenium 12C**
  - to stop the infection

# FEVER

Fever manifests itself as an abnormally high temperature, the sign of a defense mechanism of the organism.

It represents a beneficial and salutary physiological process.

It can become troublesome in some cases (e.g. convulsive attacks in children).

Fever has a certain number of characteristics:

- level of temperature;
- variability (fluctuant fever);
- duration.

## DETERMINING SYMPTOMS

- High fever 102,2°F – 103,1°F
- Moderate fever 100,4°F – 101,3°F
- Fever with insidious onset, which then becomes continuous

## PRINCIPAL MEDICINES

## HIGH FEVER WITH RAPID ONSET

**IF**
- fever related to **exposure to icy cold** (North wind) or following a **sunstroke or heat stroke**
- rosy, **strong and active** person
- thirst for small quantities of cold water
- shivering
- **no perspiration**

→ **Aconitum napellus 12C**
5 pellets 4 times a day

**Aconitum napellus** corresponds to fever with shivering.

**IF**
- high fever, sometimes **fluctuant**
- warm **congestive** face, red when lying, pale when standing
- **sweats**
- aggravation from light
- aggravation from noise

→ **Belladonna 12C**
5 pellets 4 times a day

**Belladonna** very often follows **Aconitum napellus** when the fever has set in and the person starts sweating.

## MODERATE FEVER

**IF**
- fever of 100.4°F-101.3°F, never more, with progressive onset which is the sign of a less strong and active condition than that of the two previous medicines
- **moist** skin
- **face which is sometimes pale, sometimes red** depending on the level of the fever
- congestive phenomena, tendency to epistaxis
- possibly painful dry cough

**Ferrum phosphoricum 12C**
5 pellets twice a day

## CONTINUOUS FEVER

This type of fever has fully set in and is the sign of a more serious condition of the patient.

**IF**
- continuous fever
- **thirst for large quantities of cold water**
- **dryness of the mucous membranes**
- **aggravation from the slightest movement**
- improvement with immobility

**Bryonia alba 12C**
5 pellets 4 or 5 times a day

**IF**
- high continuous fever
- shivering
- **articular pains improved by movement**
  (the person continuously turns round in bed)
- **intense thirst**
- often starts after getting **soaked by rain**
- or chill after effort, **sweat**

**Rhus toxicodendron 12C**
5 pellets 4 or 5 times a day

**IF**
- continuous fever
- **prostrated, dazed, "dim"** person
- **shivering and trembling**
- **absence of thirst**

**Gelsemium sempervirens 12C**
5 pellets 4 or 5 times a day

## SPECIALTY

- **COLDCALM®**: Adults and children 3 years and over, dissolve 2 tablets in the mouth every 2 hours up to 6 times a day

## FEVER

- **Aconitum napellus 12C**
  - high fever with rapid onset after exposure to icy cold or after heat stroke
  - no perspiration

- **Belladonna 12C**
  - high fever with rapid onset, sometimes fluctuant
  - sweats
  - congestive face

- **Ferrum phosphoricum 12C**
  - moderate fever
  - moist skin
  - face sometimes pale, sometimes red

- **Bryonia alba 12C**
  - continuous fever
  - dryness of mucous membranes
  - thirst for large quantities of cold water
  - aggravation from the slightest movement

- **Rhus toxicodendron 12C**
  - continuous high fever
  - articular pains relieved by movement
  - intense thirst

- **Gelsemium sempervirens 12C**
  - continuous fever
  - absence of thirst
  - shivering, trembling, prostration

# HAY FEVER

Hay fever is a form of spasmodic coryza related to:
- environmental factors (pollens);
- constitutional factors of the patient (allergies).

It is a form of allergic rhinitis, which also includes allergic sensitivity to dust, acarids, volatile chemical substances, etc.

Hay fever impacts the overall condition of the patient, due to its persistence and the permanent discomfort it entails (restricted breathing, loss of perception of odor and taste).

## DETERMINING SYMPTOMS
- spasmodic sneezing of a periodic nature,
- clear and fluid nasal discharge,
- ocular irritation,
- itching (nose, ears, soft palate).

## PRINCIPAL MEDICINES

**IF**
- **irritant nasal discharge burning** the upper lip (redness)
- non-irritant ocular discharge
- **improvement in cool air**

→ **Allium cepa 12C**
5 pellets 3 or 4 times a day

**IF**
- profuse non-irritant nasal discharge
- **irritant, acrid, corrosive lacrimation** with **redness of the conjunctiva** (eyelids stuck together in the morning)
- **smarting sensation** in the eyes, as from sand

→ **Euphrasia officinalis 12C**
5 pellets 3 or 4 times a day

**IF**
- **irritation of the nose and eyes**
- **much sneezing**

→ **Naphthalinum 12C**
5 pellets 3 or 4 times a day

**IF**
- profuse watery discharge
- sneezing
- spasmodic cough triggering sneezing
- thready mucus discharged from the nose

→ **Badiaga 12C**
5 pellets 3 or 4 times a day

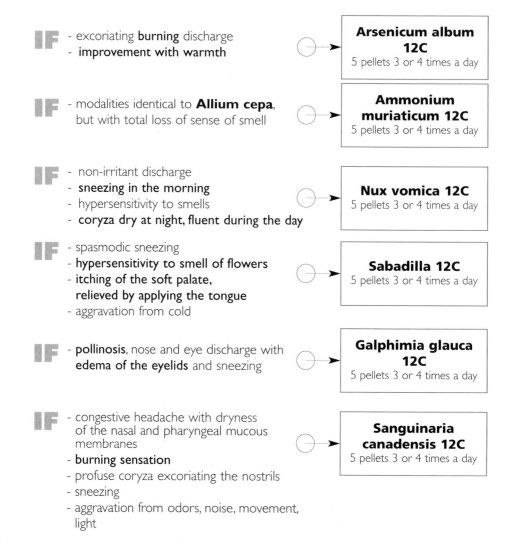

**IF**
- excoriating **burning** discharge
- **improvement with warmth**

**Arsenicum album 12C**
5 pellets 3 or 4 times a day

**IF**
- modalities identical to **Allium cepa**, but with total loss of sense of smell

**Ammonium muriaticum 12C**
5 pellets 3 or 4 times a day

**IF**
- non-irritant discharge
- **sneezing in the morning**
- hypersensitivity to smells
- **coryza dry at night, fluent during the day**

**Nux vomica 12C**
5 pellets 3 or 4 times a day

**IF**
- spasmodic sneezing
- **hypersensitivity to smell of flowers**
- **itching of the soft palate, relieved by applying the tongue**
- aggravation from cold

**Sabadilla 12C**
5 pellets 3 or 4 times a day

**IF**
- **pollinosis**, nose and eye discharge with **edema of the eyelids** and sneezing

**Galphimia glauca 12C**
5 pellets 3 or 4 times a day

**IF**
- congestive headache with dryness of the nasal and pharyngeal mucous membranes
- **burning sensation**
- profuse coryza excoriating the nostrils
- sneezing
- aggravation from odors, noise, movement, light

**Sanguinaria canadensis 12C**
5 pellets 3 or 4 times a day

## PREVENTIVE TREATMENT OF HAY FEVER

The repetition of hay fever each year calls for a preventive treatment in order to lessen the effects.

Simple recommendations from a pharmacist or a nurse will endeavor to reduce or prevent the allergic inflammatory reaction.

Individual prophylaxis must remain the responsibility of the physician (constitutional treatment and prescription of specific hetero-isothera-peutics, as well as isolation of the allergen).

## SPECIALTIES

- **SABADIL®**: For temporary relief of symptoms of hay fever or other respiratory allergies.
  Adults and children 6 years and over, dissolve 2 tablets in the mouth every 15 minutes for 1 hour, then 2 tablets 3 times a day.
- **SINUSALIA®**: For congestion and pain due to inflammation of the sinuses.
  Adults and children 6 years and over, dissolve 2 tablets in the mouth every 2 hours up to 6 times a day.
- **OPTIQUE 1®** eye drops: For minor eye irritation due to fatigue or airborne irritants such as ragweed, other pollens and dust.
  Instill 1 or 2 drops in affected eye(s). Repeat 2 to 6 times a day.

## HAY FEVER

- **Allium cepa 12C**
  - nasal discharge burning the upper lip
  - non-irritant lacrimation
  - improvement in cool air

- **Euphrasia officinalis 12C**
  - non-irritant nasal discharge
  - corrosive lacrimation
  - sensation of smarting in the eyes

- **Naphthalinum 12C**
  - much sneezing
  - irritation of the eyes and nose

- **Badiaga 12C**
  - profuse watery discharge
  - improvement with warmth, contrary to **Allium cepa**
  - sneezing

- **Arsenicum album 12C**
  - excoriating burning discharge
  - improvement with warmth

- **Ammonium muriaticum 12C**
  - modalities identical to those of Allium cepa, but with total loss of sense of smell

- **Nux vomica 12C**
  - sneezing in the morning
  - hypersensitivity to odors
  - coryza dry at night, fluent during the day

- **Sabadilla 12C**
  - spasmodic sneezing
  - hypersensitivity to odor of flowers
  - itching of the soft palate
  - aggravation from cold

- **Galphimia glauca 12C**
  - pollinosis, nose and eye discharge with edema of the eyelids and sneezing

- **Sanguinaria canadensis 12C**
  - congestive headache
  - profuse coryza, excoriating the nostrils
  - sneezing
  - aggravation from odors, noise, movement, light

# HERPES SIMPLEX (COLD SORES)

## DETERMINING SYMPTOMS

Eruption of pruritic clusters of vesicles, commonly known as cold sores fever blisters.

## PRINCIPAL MEDICINES

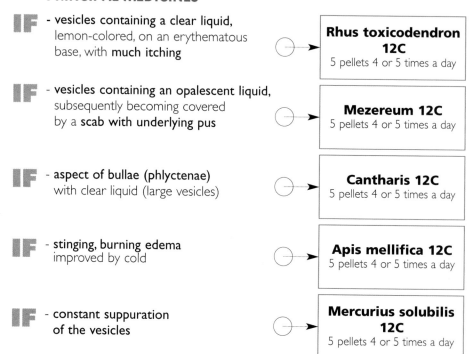

**IF** - vesicles containing a clear liquid, lemon-colored, on an erythematous base, with **much itching**

> **Rhus toxicodendron 12C**
> 5 pellets 4 or 5 times a day

**IF** - vesicles containing an opalescent liquid, subsequently becoming covered by a **scab with underlying pus**

> **Mezereum 12C**
> 5 pellets 4 or 5 times a day

**IF** - aspect of bullae (phlyctenae) with clear liquid (large vesicles)

> **Cantharis 12C**
> 5 pellets 4 or 5 times a day

**IF** - stinging, burning edema improved by cold

> **Apis mellifica 12C**
> 5 pellets 4 or 5 times a day

**IF** - constant suppuration of the vesicles

> **Mercurius solubilis 12C**
> 5 pellets 4 or 5 times a day

✔ Recurrent herpes indicates a constitutional problem, which requires a medical opinion (**Natrum muriaticum, Thuja occidentalis**).
Factors triggering a bout of herpes are very often related to exposure to the sun, vexations, tiredness.

## SPECIALTIES

- **COLD SORE CAREKIT** contains **Rhus toxicodendron 12C, Apis mellifica 12C** and **Mezereum 12C**
- **CALENDULA OINTMENT**: apply a thin layer on the lesion to moisturize and promote healing.

## HERPES SIMPLEX

- **Rhus toxicodendron 12C**
  - vesicles with clear liquid
  - itching

- **Mezereum 12C**
  - vesicles with opalescent liquid, scabs

- **Mercurius solubilis 12C**
  - vesicles + suppuration

- **Apis mellifica 12C**
  - stinging burning edema, relieved by cold

- **Cantharis 12C**
  - bullae

# HERPES ZOSTER

Herpes zoster (shingles) is characterized by the appearance on the skin of a number of small blisters on a background of red skin. It is linked to a neurotropic virus.

The pharmacist's advice should be limited to recent and circumscribed cases of zoster, in individuals whose general condition does not seem to be unduly affected.

## DETERMINING SYMPTOMS

This condition is distinguished by:
- a unilateral eruption localized along a nerve pathway (intercostal or ocular),
- a sharp, shooting neuralgic pain.

## PRINCIPAL MEDICINES

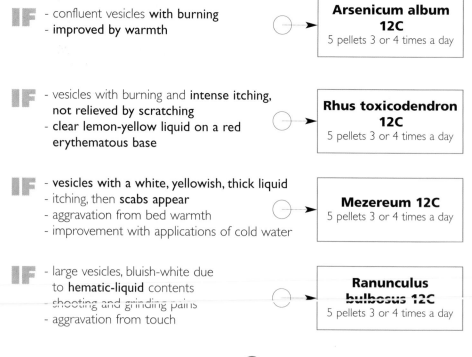

**IF**
- confluent vesicles **with burning**
- **improved by warmth**

**Arsenicum album 12C**
5 pellets 3 or 4 times a day

**IF**
- vesicles with burning and **intense itching, not relieved by scratching**
- **clear lemon-yellow liquid on a red erythematous base**

**Rhus toxicodendron 12C**
5 pellets 3 or 4 times a day

**IF**
- **vesicles with a white, yellowish, thick liquid**
- itching, then **scabs appear**
- aggravation from bed warmth
- improvement with applications of cold water

**Mezereum 12C**
5 pellets 3 or 4 times a day

**IF**
- large vesicles, bluish-white due to **hematic-liquid** contents
- shooting and grinding pains
- aggravation from touch

**Ranunculus bulbosus 12C**
5 pellets 3 or 4 times a day

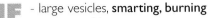
- large vesicles, **smarting, burning**
- aggravated by water
- **improved by cold**

**Cantharis 12C**
5 pellets 3 or 4 times a day

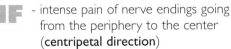
- intense pain of nerve endings going
  from the periphery to the center
  (centripetal direction)
- **aggravation from touch**
- **aggravation from jolts**

**Hypericum perforatum 30C**
5 pellets 3 or 4 times a day

The "**Arnica** of the nerves".

## HERPES ZOSTER

- **Arsenicum album 12C**
  - confluent vesicles with burning
  - improvement with warmth and warm
    applications

- **Rhus toxicodendron 12C**
  - vesicles with burning and itching not
    relieved by scratching
  - clear lemon-yellow liquid

- **Mezereum 12C**
  - vesicles with thick white liquid
  - aggravation from bed warmth
  - improvement with application
    of cold water

- **Ranunculus bulbosus 12C**
  - large vesicles
  - hematic bluish-white liquid
  - shooting and grinding pains
  - aggravation from touch

- **Cantharis 12C**
  - large burning vesicles
  - improvement with cold applications

- **Hypericum perforatum 30C**
  - intense pain of nerve endings
    (centripetal direction)
  - aggravation from touch
  - aggravation from jolts
  - "the Arnica of the nerves"

# HOT FLUSHES OF MENOPAUSE

The female menopause is characterized by the gradual disappearance of the menstrual flow.

Periods become less regular and less abundant, and finally disappear. This situation can give rise to a number of disorders, including hypertension and osteoporosis, and to frequent hot flushes, which may be experienced as more or less tolerable or as quite unbearable.

The onset of all these symptoms varies greatly from one woman to another.

## DETERMINING SYMPTOMS

The homeopathic medicine which is most commonly employed during the premenopausal and menopausal phases is **Lachesis mutus**.

The absence or delay of a physiological or pathological flow are characteristic of **Lachesis mutus** in the same way that **Cinchona officinalis** is indicated in cases of abundant or repeated loss of organic liquids.

In the premenopausal phase, the prescription of doses of **Lachesis mutus** in a rising scale (9C, 15C, and 30C on the 20th, 21st, and 22nd days of the cycle respectively) regulates the pathological disturbances during this phase.

## PRINCIPAL MEDICINES

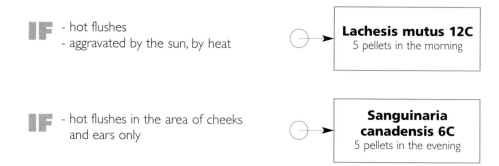

**IF**
- hot flushes
- aggravated by the sun, by heat

**Lachesis mutus 12C**
5 pellets in the morning

**IF**
- hot flushes in the area of cheeks and ears only

**Sanguinaria canadensis 6C**
5 pellets in the evening

## SPECIALTY

• **HOT FLUSHES CAREKIT** contains **Lachesis mutus 12C, Glonoinum 12C** and **Sanguinaria canadensis 12C.**

## HOT FLUSHES OF MENOPAUSE

- **Lachesis mutus 12C**
  - aggravation from the sun, from heat

- **Sanguinaria canadensis 6C**
  - red cheeks and ears

# INFLUENZA or SYMPTOMS OF FLU

## DETERMINING SYMPTOMS

To be noted:
• aches and pains,
• fever,
• headache,
• shivering.

**Frequent associated symptoms:**
- tracheobronchial irritation,
- ocular pains,
- digestive involvement (nausea - sickly feeling - diarrhea).

## PRINCIPAL MEDICINES

In all cases, to be taken as soon as possible:
• 1 unit-dose of **Oscillococcinum®**: repeat every 6 hours until improvement.

Follow with:
• 1 dose of **Sulphur 15C** only 1 hour after the last dose of **Oscillococcinum®**.

Depending on the symptoms, the following medicines will be added:

 - fever
- **prostrated, dazed, "dim"** person
- crimson face
- shivering and **trembling**
- intense fatigue
- **absence of thirst**
- headache
- **frontal headache with heaviness of the eyeballs**

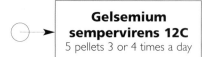

**Gelsemium sempervirens 12C**
5 pellets 3 or 4 times a day

 - fever
- **aches, articular pains relieved by movement**
- **intense thirst for cold water**
- digestive involvement with tense abdomen

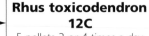

**Rhus toxicodendron 12C**
5 pellets 3 or 4 times a day

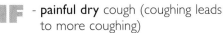 - **osseous** pains (sensation of broken bones)
- headache + **pain of the eyeballs**
  **with pressure**
- digestive involvement (**aversion for food**)
- **tracheobronchial irritation**

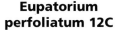

| **Eupatorium perfoliatum 12C** |
| 5 pellets 3 or 4 times a day |

- **painful dry** cough (coughing leads
  to more coughing)
- **intense thirst for cold water**
- **aggravation from movement**
- **dry mucous membranes**

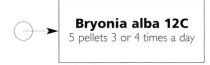

| **Bryonia alba 12C** |
| 5 pellets 3 or 4 times a day |

## SPECIALTY

• **OSCILLOCOCCINUM®** (Anas barbariae hepatic et cordis extractum 200CK), 1 unit-dose every 6 hours until improvement.

### INFLUENZA or INFLUENZAL SYMPTOMS

• **Gelsemium sempervirens 12C**
- fever
- intense fatigue
- shivering, trembling
- absence of thirst
- headache

• **Rhus toxicodendron 12C**
- fever
- aches relieved by movement
- intense thirst for cold water

• **Eupatorium perfoliatum 12C**
- osseous pains
- sensation of broken bones
- ocular pains

• **Bryonia alba 12C**
- painful dry cough
  (coughing leads to more coughing)
- dry mucous membranes
- intense thirst for cold water
- improvement with immobility
- pains in the chest

# INSECT BITES OR STINGS

The response of the organism to insect bites and stings varies depending on:
- the nature of the causative agent;
- the location;
- the sensitivity of the individual concerned (allergic reaction).

The pharmacist is often the first to be consulted; he or she must be able to respond with emergency treatment, while waiting for the doctor if necessary.

Any insect bite or sting should be disinfected with diluted mother tincture of **Calendula**, or with another suitable antiseptic, after removing the sting if necessary.


## PRINCIPAL MEDICINES

**IF** - burning stinging edema,
  relieved by applications of cold water
  (bee, wasp, horsefly, etc.)
→ **Apis mellifica 30C**
5 pellets 3 or 4 times a day

Because some subjects are particularly sensitive, for example bee-keepers who acquire a sensitivity to bee venom, high (15C) dilutions should always be given.

**IF** - cold, mottled, pale skin
- with impression of local paralysis
→ **Ledum palustre 6C**
5 pellets 3 or 4 times a day

**IF** - local tissue inflammation, with a deep red color, burning pain, induration, characteristic of a spider bite
(very often following several bites)
→ **Tarentula cubensis 6C**
5 pellets 3 or 4 times a day

**IF** - itching pains
- jellyfish stings
→ **Urtica urens 6C**
5 pellets 3 or 4 times a day

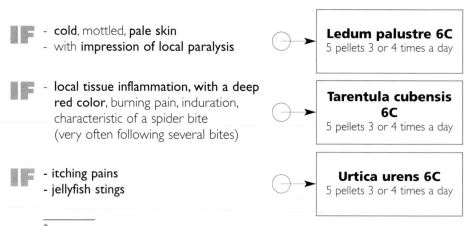

---

\* *Apis mellifica* is a mother tincture prepared from the whole bee. *Apium virus* or *Apisinum* is prepared from the venom.

Some insect bites or stings only worry the patient on the following day, when there is inflammation and red tumefaction of the skin with pain.

While waiting to see the doctor, the following can be useful:
1) compresses with rubbing alcohol;
2) **Belladonna** ("tumor – rubor – dolor – calor") 5C, 5 pellets 3 or 4 times a day;
3) **Pyrogenium 12C** to avoid infection, 5 pellets twice a day, and **Bufo rana 5C** to avoid lymphangitis, 5 pellets 3 or 4 times a day.

---

### LOCAL TREATMENT

Apply locally on insect bites or stings:
**Apis mellifica** MT ana,
**Ledum palustre** MT ana,
**Calendula** MT ana.

---

 For bites of venomous snakes, try to prevent diffusion of the venom and refer promptly to the physician or the hospital.

---

### INSECT BITES OR STINGS

- **Apis mellifica 30C**
  - stinging burning edema
  - improved by application of cold water

- **Ledum palustre 6C**
  - cold mottled skin
  - impression of local paralysis

- **Tarentula cubensis 6C**
  (spider)
  - local inflammation of tissue
  - induration

- **Belladonna 6C**
  - "tumor - rubor - dolor - calor"

- **Bufo rana 6C**
  - to avoid lymphangitis

- **Pyrogenium 12C**
  - to avoid infection

- **Urtica urens 6C**
  - jellyfish stings
  - itching pains

# MOTION SICKNESS

Motion sickness is a malaise starting with dizziness, loss of color in the face, and headache.

Nausea and very often painful vomiting follow.

Homeopathic medicines, taken preventively (5 pellets twice a day) and repeated during the journey, help diminish symptoms without inducing drowsiness.

## PRINCIPAL MEDICINES

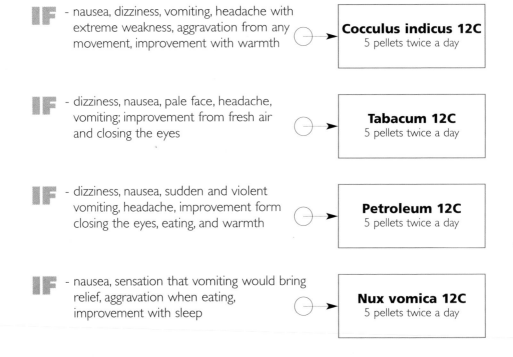

**IF** - nausea, dizziness, vomiting, headache with extreme weakness, aggravation from any movement, improvement with warmth

**Cocculus indicus 12C**
5 pellets twice a day

**IF** - dizziness, nausea, pale face, headache, vomiting; improvement from fresh air and closing the eyes

**Tabacum 12C**
5 pellets twice a day

**IF** - dizziness, nausea, sudden and violent vomiting, headache, improvement form closing the eyes, eating, and warmth

**Petroleum 12C**
5 pellets twice a day

**IF** - nausea, sensation that vomiting would bring relief, aggravation when eating, improvement with sleep

**Nux vomica 12C**
5 pellets twice a day

## SPECIALTY

- **COCCULINE**: 2 tablets 3 times a day the day before and on the day of the journey, or 1 unit-dose tube the day before and 1 just before the journey.

## MOTION SICKNESS

- **Cocculus indicus 12C**
  - nausea, dizziness, vomiting
  - aggravation from any movement

- **Tabacum 12C**
  - dizziness, nausea, pallor
  - improvement with fresh air
    and with the eyes closed

- **Petroleum 12C**
  - dizziness, nausea, violent vomiting
  - improvement from warmth, eating,
    closing the eyes

- **Nux vomica 12C**
  - nausea, sensation that vomiting
    would bring relief
  - aggravation when eating

# OTITIS

Otitis is an acute inflammation of the middle ear, occurring after a chill (from dry cold, or from bathing, etc.), or following a head cold, tonsillitis, or influenza.

## DETERMINING SYMPTOMS

Acute otitis media is of abrupt onset.
It is characterized by a violent pain in the auditory canal which rapidly becomes a throbbing pain.
It is accompanied by a raised temperature with shivering and sweating.

✔ The pharmacist can only intervene in the congestive phase.
As this phase is short, we must be able to give the appropriate homeopathic medicines very rapidly.

## PRINCIPAL MEDICINES

**IF**
- otitis with **unbearable acute pain** after sudden chill
- warm red auricle of the ear
- **dry skin**
- **high fever with rapid onset**

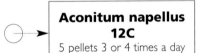

**Aconitum napellus 12C**
5 pellets 3 or 4 times a day

**IF**
- otitis with **throbbing pain**
- high fever
- **sweating**
- hypersensitivity to noise

**Belladonna 12C**
5 pellets 3 or 4 times a day

**IF**
- otitis with sharp pains
- **temperature: 100.4°F, 101.3°F**
- **moist skin**
- headache

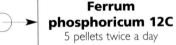

**Ferrum phosphoricum 12C**
5 pellets twice a day

**IF**
- **pains** becoming **unbearable** because of hyperesthesia to pain, especially in children, who become aggressive, irritable, **with one red and one pale cheek**
especially for otitis related to teething

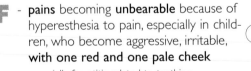

**Chamomilla 30C**
5 pellets 3 or 4 times a day

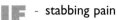 - **stabbing pain**
- aggravated by cold
- sensation of burning
  (not relieved by warmth)

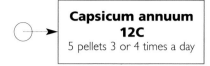

**Capsicum annuum 12C**
5 pellets 3 or 4 times a day

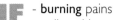 - **burning** pains
- relieved by warmth

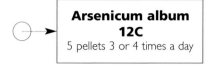

**Arsenicum album 12C**
5 pellets 3 or 4 times a day

## OTITIS

- **Aconitum napellus 12C**
  - unbearable acute pains
  - warm red auricle of the ear
  - high fever with rapid onset

- **Belladonna 12C**
  - throbbing pains
  - high fever
  - sweating
  - hypersensitivity to noises

- **Ferrum phosphoricum 12C**
  - sharp pains
  - fever: 100.4°F, 101.3°F
  - moist skin
  - headache

- **Chamomilla 30C**
  - unbearable pains in children,
    related to teething

- **Capsicum annuum 12C**
  - stabbing pain, aggravated by cold
  - sensation of burning
  - not improved by warmth

- **Arsenicum album 12C**
  - burning pains
  - relieved by warmth

# PINWORMS

Oxyuriasis is the infestation of the digestive tract by pinworms (oxyurids), which may be found in the stools.

The most common locations of pinworms within the digestive tract are around the ileocecal valve, and in the terminal segment of the intestine.

The condition is most common in children.

There is usually an exacerbation of symptoms at times of moon changes (new and full moons), which correspond to the hatching of the eggs and the release of toxins.

Certain children seem to be infested more often than others, according to a constitutional predisposition.

## Etiology

Contamination occurs principally via the fingernails and the ingestion of the eggs, hence the need for strict measures of hygiene.

Prophylactic measures include hand-washing with careful nail cleaning and changing underwear (including pajamas) daily.

### DETERMINING SYMPTOMS

Worm infestation is revealed by three types of disturbances:
- digestive disorders: bad breath, nausea, vomiting;
- nervous disorders: irritable and insomniac children, with night terrors, grinding of teeth, or convulsions;
- general disorders: coughing with constant clearing of the throat, itching (principally anal), rubbing of the nose.

## PRINCIPAL MEDICINES

In homeopathy, there are no worm-killing medicines; these may be necessary in cases of massive infestation.

**IF**  - the child is aggressive, sullen, with rings under
        the eyes
      - grinding of teeth at night
      - abdominal pains around the navel
      - urinary incontinence at night
      - itching of the anus
      - itching of the nose
      - dry cough with attempts to clear the throat

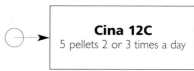

**Cina 12C**
5 pellets 2 or 3 times a day

In case of constitutional problems, **Cina** can be given in 15C, one dose per week or every other week.

**IF**  - pale face, bad breath
      - headache, palpitations

**Spigelia anthelmia 12C**
5 pellets 2 or 3 times a day

**IF**  - agitated child, who fidgets
        and constantly moves his hands;
        insomniac with nights terrors
      - aggravation with the new moon

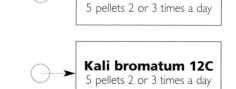

**Kali bromatum 12C**
5 pellets 2 or 3 times a day

This medicine is also indicated in cases of sleepwalking.

---

**PINWORMS**

- **Cina 12C**
  - aggressive child
  - rings under the eyes
  - abdominal pains
  - itching of the anus
  - dry cough

- **Spigelia anthelmia 12C**
  - pale face
  - bad breath
  - palpitations

- **Kali bromatum 12C**
  - agitated child
  - night fears
  - aggravated with the new moon

# PREGNANCY
# GASTRIC DISORDERS

These disorders are related to pressure on the stomach which engenders problems of reflux, hyperacidity, burning.

## PRINCIPAL MEDICINES

**IF** - acidity is predominant

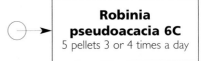

**Robinia pseudoacacia 6C**
5 pellets 3 or 4 times a day

**IF** - burning is predominant

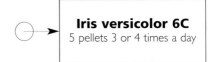

**Iris versicolor 6C**
5 pellets 3 or 4 times a day

---

### SPECIALTY

• **ACIDIL** ®: For relief of occasionnal heartburn, acid indigestion or sour stomach.
Adults and children 12 and older, at the onset of symptoms dissolve 2 tablets in the mouth and repeat if needed every 15 minutes for 3 more doses. Then if necessary take 2 tablets 15 minutes before meals.

---

### PREGNANCY: GASTRIC DISORDERS

• **Robinia pseudoacacia 6C**
- if acidity is predominant

• **Iris versicolor 6C**
- if burning is predominant

# PREGNANCY
# NAUSEA, VOMITING

## DETERMINING SYMPTOMS
Nausea, vomiting.

## PRINCIPAL MEDICINES

**IF** - nausea not relieved by vomiting, hypersalivation, **clear tongue**
and food cravings

**Ipecac 12C**
5 pellets
when the nausea occurs

**Ipecac** is used as an emetic in allopathic treatments.

**IF** - nausea triggered by the slightest smell,
improved when eating, with **hypersensitivity to vexation**

**Ignatia amara 12C**
5 pellets
when the nausea occurs

Consider **Ignatia amara** whenever pregnancy is not wanted or makes the woman ill.

**IF** - irrepressible vomiting
- hypersensitivity to cooking smells,
**craving for vinegar**, pickles, acidic food
and drink, aversion for milk

**Sepia 12C**
5 pellets
when the nausea occurs

**IF** - nausea or vomiting
- aggravated by the slightest movement,
with disgust for food

**Symphoricarpus
racemosus 12C**
5 pellets
when the nausea occurs

In case of associated vertigo, refer to medicines for motion sickness: **Cocculus
indicus, Tabacum, Petroleum,** and above all, refer to the physician.

## PREGNANCY: NAUSEA, VOMITING

- **Ipecac 12C**
  - hypersalivation
  - clear tongue
  - food cravings
  - nausea not improved by vomiting

- **Ignatia amara 12C**
  - nausea aggravated by smells, improved when eating
  - hypersensitivity to vexation

- **Sepia 12C**
  - irresistible vomiting
  - hypersensitivity to cooking smells
  - desire for vinegar, pickles
  - aversion for milk

- **Symphoricarpus racemosus 12C**
  - disgust for all foods

# PREGNANCY
# URINARY DISORDERS

Pregnant women are often prone to constipation and urinary disorders resulting from pressure on the bladder.
Above all, the urinary level of albumin should be regularly checked.

## PRINCIPAL MEDICINES

**IF**
- frequent desire to urinate
- with **sensation of pressure on the bladder**

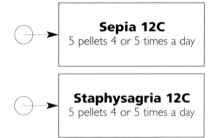

**Sepia 12C**
5 pellets 4 or 5 times a day

**IF**
- burning of the urethra between each micturition or **sensation of a drop of urine escaping** after micturition

**Staphysagria 12C**
5 pellets 4 or 5 times a day

**Staphysagria** is often indicated in urinary disorders of pregnancy when **the pregnancy is accompanied by health problems**, or where there is **touchiness, repressed emotions**, hypersensitivity to vexation.

**IF**
- pain before, during, and after micturition (cystitis)

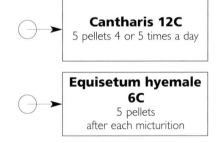

**Cantharis 12C**
5 pellets 4 or 5 times a day

**IF**
- pains after micturition

**Equisetum hyemale 6C**
5 pellets
after each micturition

---

### PREGNANCY: URINARY DISORDERS

- **Sepia 12C**
  - frequent desire to urinate
  - with sensation of pressure on the bladder

- **Staphysagria 12C**
  - burning of the urethra between each micturition
  - or sensation of a drop of urine escaping after micturition

- **Cantharis 12C**
  - pain before, during, and after micturition (cystitis)

- **Equisetum hyemale 6C**
  - pains after micturition

# RHEUMATIC PAIN

The dispensing pharmacist cannot treat chronic rheumatism.

Acute rheumatic fever, characterized by fever, inflammation, and redness is considered to be an infectious disease; it is imperative to consult a physician (cardiac complications are possible).

Chronic rheumatism is a common disease, evolving in successive bouts; it can lead to articular deformation, restricted movement, and progressive ankylosis.

From an etiological point of view, chronic rheumatism is linked to constitutional factors, poor diet (leading to metabolic problems), and age-related "wearing down".

Chronic rheumatism is generally aggravated by cold and damp, which are factors causing vasoconstriction.

Patients must consult a physician.

Allopathic treatment is mainly based on sedation of pain with analgesics such as aspirin, or on anti-inflammatory drugs.

This type of therapy may give rise to problems of intolerance: long-term treatment often leads to gastric or colonic problems.

Pharmacists or nurses can give appropriate advice to follow or to accompany allopathic treatment, enabling the doses of more aggressive drugs to be reduced.

## DETERMINING SYMPTOMS

The health care professional should seek primarily to establish the modalities of appearance or sedation of pain:
- links to movement or absence of movement;
- links to atmospheric conditions, cold, damp, heat, wind, storms, etc.

## PRINCIPAL MEDICINES

Advice given by the pharmacist can only concern symptomatic relief. In acute therapeutics, some homeopathic medicines assist in the sedation of pain.

**IF** 
- rheumatic pains with muscular and articular **morning stiffness**
- **relieved by slow and progressive movement**, stiffness recurring at the end of the day
- relieved by warmth and warm applications
- **improvement in dry and hot weather**

**Rhus toxicodendron 12C**
5 pellets twice a day

**IF**
- dull rheumatic pains, **more muscular than articular**
- aggravated by humidity
- improved by dry weather, movement

**Dulcamara 12C**
5 pellets twice a day

**IF**
- articular stiffness, muscular contractions
- aggravated by dry cold
- **improved by damp rainy weather and by warmth**

**Causticum 12C**
5 pellets twice a day

**IF**
- rheumatic pains
- **aggravated before a storm and by static electricity in the air**
- improved after the storm by dry warmth, by movement

**Rhododendron chrysanthum 12C**
5 pellets twice a day

**IF**
- rheumatic pains with **red, shiny, stiff, swollen joints; pains as from red-hot needles**
- aggravated by warmth, touch, pressure, movement
- improved by rest, by **cold applications**

**Apis mellifica 12C**
5 pellets twice a day

**IF**
- rheumatic pains with **general stiffness and aches**
- **aggravated by the slightest touch**, cold, **movement**
- **improved by rest**, lying with the head low

**Arnica montana 12C**
5 pellets twice a day

**IF** - rheumatic pains
- **aggravated by the slightest movement** or touch
- **improved by rest, strong pressure,** when lying on the painful side

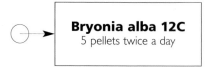

**Bryonia alba 12C**
5 pellets twice a day

**IF** - **rheumatism of the small joints,** wrists, **joints of the fingers**
- **interphalangeal deformation**

• **first phalanx, extremities**

**Actaea spicata 3X**
20 drops twice a day

• **all phalanges**

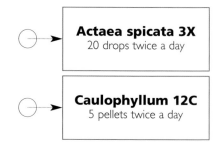

**Caulophyllum 12C**
5 pellets twice a day

Judicious homeopathic treatments, combined with treatment with trace elements (Mn Cu, Mn Co, etc.), as well as phytotherapy, make it possible to improve the condition of patients suffering from rheumatism and to extend the range of possible movement, and thus to limit the onset of progressive ankylosis, without negative effects on the digestive tract.

## SPECIALTIES

• **ARNICALM ARTHRITIS®** for temporary relief of minor aches and pains associated with arthritis.
Adults and children 12 years and over, dissolve 5 pellets in the mouth 3 times a day.
• **ARNICA CREAM**, apply a thin layer to affected area and massage gently 3 times a day.

## RHEUMATIC PAIN

• **Rhus toxicodendron 12C**
- pains with muscular and articular stiffness in the morning
- improvement with slow and progressive movement, with warm applications

• **Dulcamara 12C**
- dull muscular pains
- aggravation from humidity
- improvement in dry weather and movement

• **Causticum 12C**
- articular stiffness
- muscular contractions
- improvement in humid weather, with warmth
- aggravation from dry cold

• **Rhododendron chrysanthum 12C**
- rheumatic pains
- aggravation before a storm
- improvement after the storm, with dry heat, with movement

- **Apis mellifica 12C**
  - pains with swollen joints
  - pains as from burning needles
  - aggravation from warmth, pressure, movement
  - improvement with cold applications, with rest

- **Arnica montana 12C**
  - pains with stiffness and general aches
  - aggravation from movement, from cold
  - improvement with rest

- **Bryonia alba 12C**
  - pains with aggravation from the slightest movement or contact
  - improvement with rest, lying on the painful side

- **Actaea spicata 3X**
  - rheumatism of the small joints
  - deformation of the first phalanx

- **Caulophyllum 12C**
  - rheumatism of the small joints
  - interphalangeal deformation

# SORE THROAT

The pharmacist can only give advice for sore throat of **sudden and recent onset**, accompanying an inflammation related to a chill, or in the context of an influenza epidemic.

## DETERMINING SYMPTOMS

As it is not possible for the heath care professional to make a direct assessment of the inflammation, the determining symptoms to be borne in mind are the following:
- etiology;
- nature of the pain;
- specific sensations;
- localization as defined by the patient;
- accompanying general signs (fever).

 Pharmacists or nurses can only intervene on an ad-hoc basis. If there is no rapid improvement, refer systematically to the physician.

## PRINCIPAL MEDICINES

**IF**
- pain with sensation of throbbing
- sensation of local heat
- **dryness of the mucous membranes**
- fever with sweating

→ **Belladonna 12C**
5 pellets 3 or 4 times a day

**IF**
- hypersalivation
- thick **yellowish tongue**
  (retaining lateral teethmarks)
- fetid breath

→ **Mercurius solubilis 12C**
5 pellets 3 or 4 times a day

**IF**
- sharp pain **radiating to the ears and neck when swallowing**
- **general aches and pains**

→ **Phytolacca decandra 12C**
5 pellets 3 or 4 times a day

**IF**
- pain located on the **left,** often shifting to the right
- **difficulty swallowing liquids,** especially hot liquids

→ **Lachesis mutus 12C**
5 pellets once a day

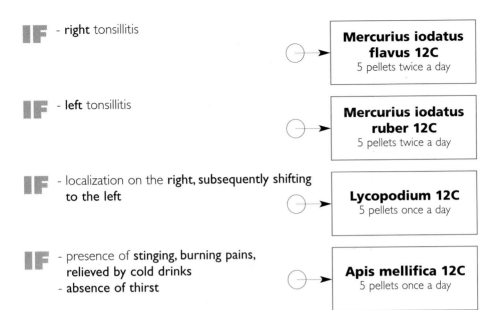

**IF** - **right** tonsillitis → **Mercurius iodatus flavus 12C**
5 pellets twice a day

**IF** - **left** tonsillitis → **Mercurius iodatus ruber 12C**
5 pellets twice a day

**IF** - localization on the **right, subsequently shifting to the left** → **Lycopodium 12C**
5 pellets once a day

**IF** - presence of **stinging, burning pains, relieved by cold drinks**
- **absence of thirst** → **Apis mellifica 12C**
5 pellets once a day

✔ The role of pharmacists is to systematically intervene in all requests for self-medication. Special attention should be paid to recurring sore throat and tonsillitis and to their persistence (hoarseness). In such cases, medical diagnosis is necessary as sore throat is often the beginning of a more severe general condition (eruptive diseases such as scarlatina, acute rheumatic fever, mononucleosis, nephritis).

## SPECIALTIES

- **ROXALIA** ® : Adults and children 12 and over, dissolve 2 tablets in the mouth every 2 hours up to 6 times a day. Children under 12: ask a doctor.
- Gargling with **Phytolacca decandra** MT and **Calendula** MT ana, 1/2 teaspoonful in a glass of warm water.

## SORE THROAT

- **Belladonna 12C**
  - "tumor - rubor - dolor - calor"
  - sweating
- **Mercurius solubilis 12C**
  - fetid breath
  - tongue retaining teethmarks
  - hypersalivation

- **Phytolacca decandra 12C**
  - sharp pains radiating to the ears and neck
  - aches and pains

- **Lachesis mutus 12C**
  - pain on the left, then shifting to the right
  - difficulty swallowing hot liquids

- **Mercurius iodatus flavus 12C**
  - right tonsillitis

- **Mercurius iodatus ruber 12C**
  - left tonsillitis

- **Lycopodium 12C**
  - pain on the right, shifting to the left

- **Apis mellifica 12C**
  - stinging, burning pains
  - relieved by cold drinks
  - absence of thirst

# STAGE FRIGHT - APPREHENSION

## DETERMINING SYMPTOMS
Loss of confidence and incapacity when faced with unusually demanding situations, such as examinations, sports competitions, stage performance.

## PRINCIPAL MEDICINES

### 1) Preparatory treatment
Should be started 2 to 4 weeks before the anxiety-producing event.

**IF**
- **loss of confidence**, numbing and slowing of mental capacity, sensation of being on a cloud
- impossible to concentrate
- shaking and loss of faculties leading to "**paralysis**" when faced with an ordeal
  the student hands in a blank script,
  a driving test candidate cannot start

→ **Gelsemium sempervirens 12C**
5 pellets a day

**IF**
- **agitation, hurried feeling**, fear of non-achievement with difficulty organizing one's ideas and great desire to get things over and done with
  the student writes the conclusion before the introduction,
  or goes off the subject from the start

→ **Argentum nitricum 12C**
5 pellets a day

**IF**
- **spasms**, lump in the throat
- **hypersensitivity** to upsets
- **hyperesthesia**
- insomnia
- **paradoxical** and contradictory symptoms

→ **Ignatia amara 12C**
5 pellets at bedtime

In practice, it is possible to give 5 pellets of **Gelsemium sempervirens 12C** a day or 5 pellets of **Argentum nitricum 12C** a day (or even both) for one month before exams are due to start, and one dose of **Gelsemium sempervirens 30C** once a week (every morning during the actual exam period). Simultaneously, in cases of loss of sleep, worry, anxiety, 5 pellets of **Ignatia**

Simultaneously, in cases of loss of sleep, worry, anxiety, 5 pellets of **Ignatia amara 12C** at bedtime.

It should also be remembered that taking 5 pellets of **Ignatia amara 12C** one hour before an oral presentation helps to release the lump in the throat characteristic of this situation.

## 2) Specific cases

**IF** - taking a driving test
- performing on stage

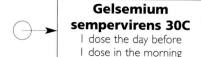

**Gelsemium sempervirens 30C**
1 dose the day before
1 dose in the morning

### SPECIALTIES

- **SEDALIA** ® : Adults and children 12 years of age and older, dissolve 2 tablets in the mouth 3 times a day.
- **STRESS CAREKIT** contains **Argentum nitricum 30C**, **Ignatia amara 30C** and **Gelsemium sempervirens 30C**

### STAGE FRIGHT — APPREHENSION

- **Gelsemium sempervirens 12C (multi-dose tube) and 30C (unit-dose tube)**
  - anticipation anxiety + "paralysis"

- **Argentum nitricum 12C**
  - hastiness

- **Ignatia amara 12C**
  - lump in the throat

# STRESS

Stress is a condition of the organism in response to emotional or physical factors. It is characterized by an exaggeration or an inhibition of the defensive mechanisms of the organism when faced with stimuli which cannot be controlled.

It can be conscious or unconscious, and can lead to excitability or to passivity.

## DETERMINING SYMPTOMS

aerophagia - allergic reactions - alopecia areata  - anxiety - aphonia - colonopathy - cramps - gastric ulceration - intermittent tetany - irritability - mental confusion - migraine - nervousness - panic attacks - sensation of constriction - sensation of exhaustion - tinnitus — trembling

## PRINCIPAL MEDICINES

**IF**
- hyperexcitability to stimuli leading to excessive irritability
- intolerance of the slightest obstacle
- aggressiveness compensated by excessive eating or drinking (coffee, alcohol, stimulants, etc.)

→ **Nux vomica 12 or 30C**
5 pellets once or twice a day

**Nux vomica** corresponds to an inappropriate response to stress that leads to more stress.

**IF**
- stress with paradoxical reactions (no apparent link of cause and effect)
- hyperesthesia, hypersensitivity to emotions, hyperemotivity
- improvement with distraction

→ **Ignatia amara 12C**
5 pellets once or twice a day

It seems that **Ignatia amara** modifies the threshold of sensitivity to stress.

**IF**
- stress dominated by fear of "non-achievement"

→ **Argentum nitricum 12C**
5 pellets once or twice a day

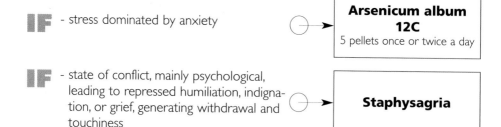

**IF** - stress dominated by anxiety ⟶ **Arsenicum album 12C**
5 pellets once or twice a day

**IF** - state of conflict, mainly psychological, leading to repressed humiliation, indignation, or grief, generating withdrawal and touchiness ⟶ **Staphysagria**

If the cause is remote in time, **Staphysagria 30C**, 5 pellets a day, increasing interval with improvement.

If the cause is recent, on 3 consecutive mornings 1 unit-dose in a scale, respectively in 6, 12, and 30C, followed by 1 weekly unit-dose in 30C, increasing interval with improvement.

## SPECIALTIES

- **SEDALIA** ® : Nervousness, hypersensivity and irritability due to stress. Adults and children 12 years of age and older, dissolve 2 tablets in the mouth 3 times a day.
- **QUIETUDE®** : sleeplessness or restless sleep. Adults and children 12 years and over, 2 tablets in the evening and 2 tablets at bedtime.
- **STRESS CAREKIT** contains **Argentum nitricum 30C, Ignatia amara 30C** and **Gelsemium sempervirens 30C**.

## STRESS

- **Nux vomica 12 or 30C**
  - hyperexcitability to stimuli leading to excessive irritability
  - intolerance of the slightest obstacle
  - aggressiveness compensated by excessive eating or drinking

- **Ignatia amara 12C**
  - stress with paradoxical reactions
  - hyperesthesia, hypersensitivity to emotions, hyperemotivity
  - improvement with distraction

- **Argentum nitricum 12C**
  - stress dominated by fear of "non-achievement"

- **Arsenicum album 12C**
  - stress dominated by anxiety

- **Staphysagria 30C**
  - state of psychological conflict leading to repressed humiliation, indignation, or grief, generating withdrawal and touchiness

# STYES - CHALAZIA

A stye is an inflammation of one of the sebaceous glands on the margin of the upper or lower eyelid.
A chalazion is a hard and painful red tumefaction of the inner eyelid.

## PRINCIPAL MEDICINES

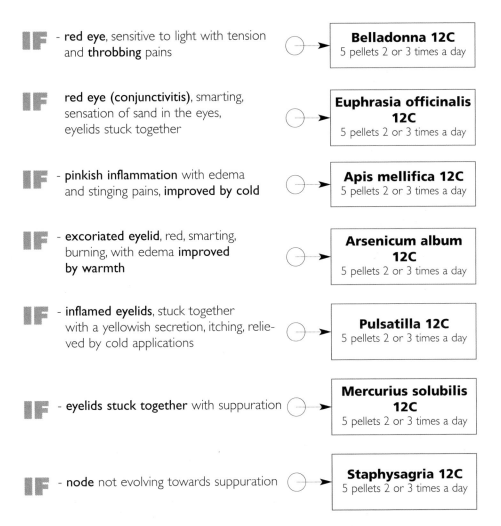

**IF** - red eye, sensitive to light with tension and **throbbing** pains

> **Belladonna 12C**
> 5 pellets 2 or 3 times a day

**IF** red eye (conjunctivitis), smarting, sensation of sand in the eyes, eyelids stuck together

> **Euphrasia officinalis 12C**
> 5 pellets 2 or 3 times a day

**IF** - pinkish inflammation with edema and stinging pains, **improved by cold**

> **Apis mellifica 12C**
> 5 pellets 2 or 3 times a day

**IF** - excoriated eyelid, red, smarting, burning, with edema **improved by warmth**

> **Arsenicum album 12C**
> 5 pellets 2 or 3 times a day

**IF** - inflamed eyelids, stuck together with a yellowish secretion, itching, relieved by cold applications

> **Pulsatilla 12C**
> 5 pellets 2 or 3 times a day

**IF** - eyelids stuck together with suppuration

> **Mercurius solubilis 12C**
> 5 pellets 2 or 3 times a day

**IF** - node not evolving towards suppuration

> **Staphysagria 12C**
> 5 pellets 2 or 3 times a day

✔ **Staphysagria** is the principal medicine for chalazia. If no positive results are obtained, refer to the ophthalmologist.

## SPECIALTY

• **OPTIQUE 1**® eye drops: 1 or 2 drops in affected eye(s). Repeat 2 to 6 times a day.

## STYES - CHALAZIA

• **Belladonna 12C**
- red eye
- throbbing pains

• **Euphrasia officinalis 12C**
- red eye
- sensation of sand in the eyes
- eyelids stuck together

• **Apis mellifica 12C**
- pinkish inflammation
- edema
- improved by cold

• **Arsenicum album 12C**
- red, burning, excoriated eyelid
- improved by warmth

• **Pulsatilla 12C**
- inflamed eyelids, stuck together with yellowish secretions
- itching

• **Mercurius solubilis 12C**
- eyelids stuck together with suppuration

• **Staphysagria 12C**
- node not evolving towards suppuration (chalazion)

# SUNSTROKE - HEAT STROKE

These terms are often confused.

**Sunstroke** is directly related to **exposure to the sun** and may therefore lead to **cutaneous burns**.

**Heat stroke** is directly related to **prolonged exposure** to heat, for example confinement in an overheated atmosphere, as in a car left in the sun. There are therefore no cutaneous burns.

## DETERMINING SYMPTOMS

**Common points of these two conditions:**
- cephalic congestion,
- shivering,
- hyperthermia,
- blocked digestion ± vomiting.

In more advance conditions, the following can be seen:
- dazed condition,
- delirium,
- loss of consciousness,
- signs of dehydration.

 **While waiting for the doctor:**
- get the person out of the sun or the heat;
- lay the person down in a cool environment, with the head downwards;
- loosen clothes;
- sprinkle the face with fresh water;
- get the person to drink slowly;
- fan the person.

## PRINCIPAL MEDICINES

- sudden **high** hyperthermia
- burning head: red face when lying, pale when standing
- thirst
- **no perspiration**
- agitation
- **anxiety, fear of dying**

| **Aconitum napellus 12C** |
| --- |
| 5 pellets 4 or 5 times a day |

- sudden hyperthermia, **high** but **fluctuant**
- crimson face
- **sweating**
- hypersensitivity to light, noise, jolts

| **Belladonna 12C** |
| --- |
| 5 pellets 4 or 5 times a day |

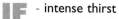 - **congestion of the head** with hot flushes and sensation of **bursting**
- red and hot face
- **red-veined eyes**, red and prominent
- **sensation of throbbing** and pulsations (temporal vein, carotid artery)
- **fixed, dazed stare**
- improvement with coolness and cold applications

**Glonoinum 12C**
5 pellets 4 or 5 times a day

 - **intense thirst**
- **aggravation from any movement**

**Bryonia alba 12C**
5 pellets 4 or 5 times a day

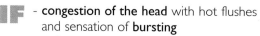 - fever
- **trembling**
- diplopia
- **absence of thirst**

**Gelsemium sempervirens 12C**
5 pellets 4 or 5 times a day

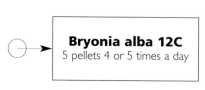
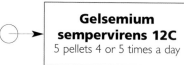

---

### SUNSTROKE - HEAT STROKE

• **Aconitum napellus 12C**
  - sudden hyperthermia
  - no perspiration
  - agitation
  - anxiety

• **Belladonna 12C**
  - sudden hyperthermia
  - sweating
  - hypersensitivity to light, noise

• **Glonoinum 12C**
  - congestion of the head
  - sensation of bursting improved by cold applications

• **Bryonia alba 12C**
  - intense thirst
  - aggravation from the slightest movement

• **Gelsemium sempervirens 12C**
  - absence of thirst
  - trembling

# SURGICAL INTERVENTIONS

The dominant features of surgical interventions are anxiety and traumatism.

Certain medicines can prepare the patient for the intervention and its after-effects.

## PRINCIPAL MEDICINES

● *Preparation before the intervention*

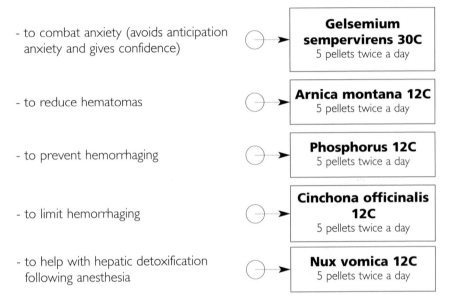

- to combat anxiety (avoids anticipation anxiety and gives confidence)

**Gelsemium sempervirens 30C**
5 pellets twice a day

- to reduce hematomas

**Arnica montana 12C**
5 pellets twice a day

- to prevent hemorrhaging

**Phosphorus 12C**
5 pellets twice a day

- to limit hemorrhaging

**Cinchona officinalis 12C**
5 pellets twice a day

- to help with hepatic detoxification following anesthesia

**Nux vomica 12C**
5 pellets twice a day

These medicines can be started one week before the intervention, 5 pellets of each twice a day.

---

● *After-effects of surgical intervention*

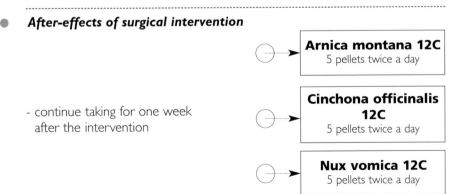

**Arnica montana 12C**
5 pellets twice a day

- continue taking for one week after the intervention

**Cinchona officinalis 12C**
5 pellets twice a day

**Nux vomica 12C**
5 pellets twice a day

- to help with cicatrization
  of clean scalpel wounds

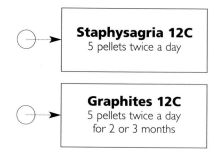

**Staphysagria 12C**
5 pellets twice a day

- in case of keloid scars (rolls)
  as soon as they appear

**Graphites 12C**
5 pellets twice a day
for 2 or 3 months

## SPECIALTIES

- **CALENDULA** ointment : apply a thin layer, once or twice a day or as needed
- **ARNICA GEL,** apply a thin layer to reduce swelling and bruising after surgery. Do not apply directly on wounds or damaged skin.
- **SEDALIA** ® : Adults and children 12 years of age and older, dissolve 2 tablets in the mouth 3 times a day.

## SURGICAL INTERVENTIONS

### PREPARATION

- **Gelsemium sempervirens 30C**
  - to combat anxiety

- **Arnica montana 12C**
  - to reduce hematomas

- **Phosphorus 12C**
  - to prevent hemorrhaging

- **Cinchona officinalis 12C**
  - to reduce hemorrhaging

- **Nux vomica 12C**
  - to help with hepatic detoxification following anesthesia

### AFTER-EFFECTS OF SURGERY

- **Arnica montana 12C**
  - continue taking for one week after surgery
- **Cinchona officinalis 12C**
  - continue taking for one week after surgery
- **Nux vomica 12C**
  - continue taking for one week after surgery

- **Staphysagria 12C**
  - helps with cicatrization of clean scalpel wounds
- **Graphites 12C**
  Calendula ointment locally
  - in case of keloid scars, as soon as they appear

# TORTICOLLIS

Torticollis (etymologically, "twisted neck") is caused by a retraction of the sternocleidomastoid muscle.

This retraction leads to a twisting of the neck muscles with the head inclined to one side, pain, and restricted movement.

Causes include drafts, chills, or a poor sleeping position.

## DETERMINING SYMPTOMS
- pain when attempting to turn the head;
- stiffness and contraction limiting rotational movement;
- head tipped to one side.

## PRINCIPAL MEDICINES

**IF**
- painful contracture and **stiffness of the sternocleidomastoid muscle**
- aggravated by rotational movement
- right laterality

→ **Lachnanthes 6C**
5 pellets 3 or 4 times a day

**IF**
- stiffness following **getting wet** (sweating from exertion)
- **improved by slow and progressive movement**

→ **Rhus toxicodendron 12C**
5 pellets 3 or 4 times a day

**IF**
- pain in the nape of the neck, compelling the person to hold the head pulled back
- tension pain in the cervical or the first dorsal vertebrae
- pain along the arms with numbing

→ **Cimicifuga racemosa 12C**
5 pellets 3 or 4 times a day

These three medicines can be combined with **Arnica montana 12C**, 5 pellets 3 or 4 times a day.

## SPECIALTIES

- **ARNICA CREAM**, apply a thin layer to affected area and massage gently 3 times a day.
- **ARNICALM® ARTHRITIS**, 5 pellets 3 times a day.

## TORTICOLLIS

- **Lachnanthes 6C**
  - painful contracture neck and shoulder blades
  - aggravated by rotational movement
  - right laterality

- **Rhus toxicodendron 12C**
  - stiffness after getting wet
  - improvement with slow movements

- **Cimicifuga racemosa 12C**
  - pain in the nape of the neck
  - improvement when holding the head back
  - pains in the cervical vertebrae

- **Arnica montana 12C**
  - in all cases

# TRAUMATISM

Traumatism is a condition resulting from an external aggression to the organism. The notion of traumatism is often limited to a sudden and accidental local lesion, but it can also be linked to repetitive actions (e.g. microtrauma, such as tendinitis).

All types of traumatism must be quantified as to their intensity and analyzed in terms of their location.

When the pharmacist is consulted first, homeopathic medication for trauma must be considered as "first aid" treatment.

The patient must subsequently be treated by a doctor.

## DETERMINING SYMPTOMS

These are to be observed visually:
• location,
• appearance,
• visible reactive modalities,
• mobility or lack of mobility,
• hemorrhaging.

The subjective appreciation of the patient is also important: nature and intensity of the pain, urge to vomit, memory of the accident.

## PRINCIPAL MEDICINES

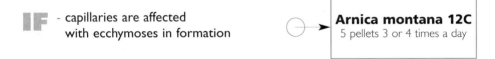

**IF** - capillaries are affected
with ecchymoses in formation → **Arnica montana 12C**
5 pellets 3 or 4 times a day

To avoid bruising, use as soon as possible.

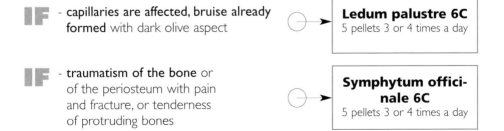

**IF** - capillaries are affected, bruise already
formed with dark olive aspect → **Ledum palustre 6C**
5 pellets 3 or 4 times a day

**IF** - traumatism of the bone or
of the periosteum with pain
and fracture, or tenderness
of protruding bones → **Symphytum officinale 6C**
5 pellets 3 or 4 times a day

This can also be used when fractures are slow to heal, in low dilution (6X), in combination with **Calcarea phosphorica 12C**, 5 pellets twice a day for a month.

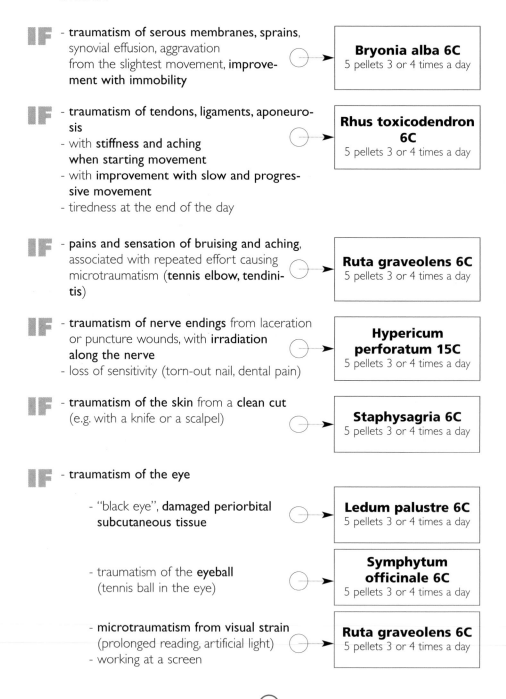

**IF** - traumatism of serous membranes, sprains, synovial effusion, aggravation from the slightest movement, **improvement with immobility**
→ **Bryonia alba 6C**
5 pellets 3 or 4 times a day

**IF** - traumatism of tendons, ligaments, aponeurosis
- with **stiffness and aching when starting movement**
- with **improvement with slow and progressive movement**
- tiredness at the end of the day
→ **Rhus toxicodendron 6C**
5 pellets 3 or 4 times a day

**IF** - **pains and sensation of bruising and aching**, associated with repeated effort causing microtraumatism (**tennis elbow, tendinitis**)
→ **Ruta graveolens 6C**
5 pellets 3 or 4 times a day

**IF** - **traumatism of nerve endings** from laceration or puncture wounds, with **irradiation along the nerve**
- loss of sensitivity (torn-out nail, dental pain)
→ **Hypericum perforatum 15C**
5 pellets 3 or 4 times a day

**IF** - **traumatism of the skin** from a **clean cut** (e.g. with a knife or a scalpel)
→ **Staphysagria 6C**
5 pellets 3 or 4 times a day

**IF** - **traumatism of the eye**

- "**black eye**", **damaged periorbital subcutaneous tissue**
→ **Ledum palustre 6C**
5 pellets 3 or 4 times a day

- traumatism of the **eyeball** (tennis ball in the eye)
→ **Symphytum officinale 6C**
5 pellets 3 or 4 times a day

- **microtraumatism from visual strain** (prolonged reading, artificial light)
- working at a screen
→ **Ruta graveolens 6C**
5 pellets 3 or 4 times a day

**IF** - traumatism with aching sensation, sensitivity to touch, little or no bruising, localization in the breast or the coccyx

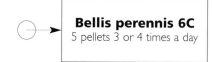

**Bellis perennis 6C**
5 pellets 3 or 4 times a day

## SPECIALTIES

- **ARNICA GEL**, apply a thin layer to affected area.
  Gel is quickly absorbed.
- **ARNICA** ointment, apply a thin layer to affected area.
  Ointment provides prologed action on sprains.
- **ARNICA CREAM**, apply a thin layer to affected area.
- **CALENDULA** ointment, apply to minor cuts and wounds, to burns and eroded skin.

## TRAUMATISM

- **Arnica montana 12C**
  - all types of traumatism

- **Ledum palustre 6C**
  - bruises already formed
  - black eye

- **Symphytum officinale 6C**
  - tennis ball in the eye

- **Bryonia alba 6C**
  - synovial effusion

- **Rhus toxicodendron 6C**
  - tendons
  - ligaments

- **Ruta graveolens 6C**
  - tendinitis
  - visual strain

- **Hypericum perforatum 30C**
  - nerve endings (teeth)

- **Staphysagria 6C**
  - clean cuts

- **Bellis perennis 6C**
  - traumatism with aching sensation, little or no bruising

# VACCINATIONS

Classical treatment to prevent possible complications: **Thuja occiden-talis** and **Sulphur**.

1 unit-dose of **Thuja occidentalis 12C** before the vaccination;

1 unit-dose of **Sulphur 12C** 48 hours after the vaccination.

# VARICOSE VEINS

A feeling of heaviness in the legs is the consequence of venous stasis. There can also be accompanying varicose veins: a permanent dilation of the veins with loss in elasticity and alteration of the walls.

This condition is usually aggravated by heat and by standing with little movement, and may be accompanied by edema, especially of the ankles at the end of the day, due to slowing of the venous return.

Venous insufficiency is very often the cause of cramps, especially at night.

Pregnant women are likely to develop varicose veins, because of compression of the venous return.

## DETERMINING SYMPTOMS
- feeling of heaviness in the legs,
- tingling,
- cramps,
- varicose veins (violaceous ecchymoses).

Phlebitis is to be suspected in case of any local or general induration of the leg with pain; refer to the physician for diagnosis and treatment.

## PRINCIPAL MEDICINES

**IF**
- feeling of heaviness in the legs with **bursting pains**
- aggravation in a vertical position
- **improvement with the legs higher up**

→ **Vipera berus 12C**
5 pellets twice a day

**IF**
- feeling of heaviness in the legs with sensation of **bruising, ecchymoses,** painful varicose veins

→ **Arnica montana 12C**
5 pellets twice a day

**IF**
- **edema** of the leg with **sensation of burning**
- **improved by cold applications**

→ **Apis mellifica 12C**
5 pellets twice a day

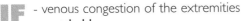

- venous congestion of the extremities
- mottled legs
- aggravation from heat
- improvement with rest, with fresh air

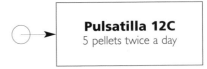

**Pulsatilla 12C**
5 pellets twice a day

Two useful drainage medicines for varicose veins, in low dilution: **Hamamelis** and **Aesculus 6X** ana, 20 drops 3 times a day.

To be noted: two medicines for the venous tissue likely to counter loss in elasticity of the supporting tissues:

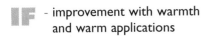

- improvement with warmth
  and warm applications

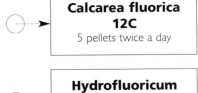

**Calcarea fluorica 12C**
5 pellets twice a day

- aggravation from heat
- improvement with cold applications

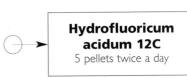

**Hydrofluoricum acidum 12C**
5 pellets twice a day

The fluorine radical is part of the composition of elastic fibers.

## SPECIALTY

- **AVENOC®** tablets, ointment or suppositories for minor symptoms of hemorrhoids such as soreness, itching and burning.

## VARICOSE VEINS

- **Vipera berus 12 C**
  - bursting pains
  - improvement with legs raised
  - aggravation when standing

- **Arnica montana 12C**
  - sensation of bruising
  - ecchymoses
  - painful varicose veins

- **Apis mellifica 12C**
  - edema of the leg with sensation of burning
  - improvement with cold applications

- **Pulsatilla 12C**
  - venous congestion of the extremities
  - mottled legs
  - improvement with rest, fresh air
  - aggravation from heat

### IN ALL CASES, ADD

- **Hamamelis 6X ana**
  20 drops 3 times a day

- **Aesculus 6X ana**
  20 drops 3 times a day

# WARTS

Warts are unpleasant and unsightly cutaneous formations.

The following should be assessed:

- localization,
- color,
- consistence.

The principal medicine for warts is **Thuja occidentalis,** one unit-dose a week in **30C**, in combination with the following medicines:

## PRINCIPAL MEDICINES

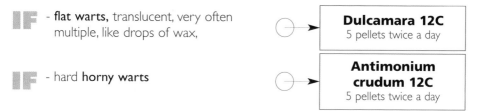

**IF** - **flat warts,** translucent, very often multiple, like drops of wax,

> **Dulcamara 12C**
> 5 pellets twice a day

**IF** - hard **horny warts**

> **Antimonium crudum 12C**
> 5 pellets twice a day

This is the medicine for plantar warts, in particular.

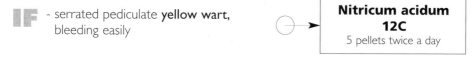

**IF** - serrated pediculate **yellow wart,** bleeding easily

> **Nitricum acidum 12C**
> 5 pellets twice a day

Often used with **Antimonium crudum** in plantar warts.

Depending on the localization, add

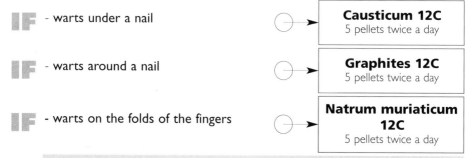

**IF** - warts under a nail

> **Causticum 12C**
> 5 pellets twice a day

**IF** - warts around a nail

> **Graphites 12C**
> 5 pellets twice a day

**IF** - warts on the folds of the fingers

> **Natrum muriaticum 12C**
> 5 pellets twice a day

## SPECIALTY

- **THUJA** ointment, wash the area, soak the wart with warm water for 5 minutes, dry thoroughly and apply a thin layer of ointment twice a day, morning and evening, for up to 12 weeks.

## WARTS

- **Thuja occidentalis 30C**
  - in all cases

- **Dulcamara 12C**
  - flat translucent warts

- **Antimonium crudum 12C**
  - hard horny warts (plantar warts)

- **Nitricum acidum 12C**
  - yellow serrated warts, bleeding easily

### DEPENDING ON LOCALIZATION

- **Causticum 12C**
  - warts under a nail

- **Graphites 12C**
  - warts around a nail

- **Natrum muriaticum 12C**
  - warts on the folds of the fingers

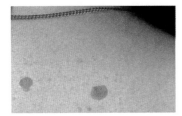

flat warts
**Dulcamara 12C**

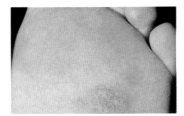

horny warts
**Antimonium crudum 12C**

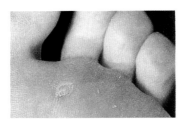

yellow warts
**Nitricum acidum 12C**

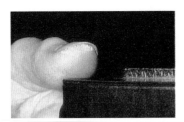

warts under a nail
**Causticum 12C**

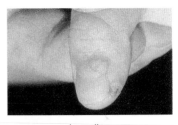

warts around a nail
**Graphites 12C**

# MATERIA MEDICA

## Homeopathic Drugs
## and their Symptomatology

# ABIES NIGRA

Black spruce
Conifers

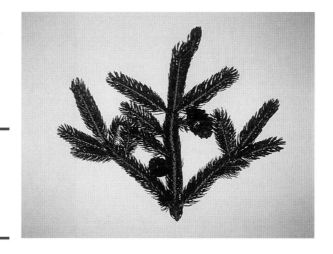

## Spasms

---

**Spasms of the esophagus and the cardia** with the sensation of a foreign body in the chest or the stomach, provoking coughing. Hiatal hernia.

# ACONITUM NAPELLUS

Aconite
Ranunculaceae

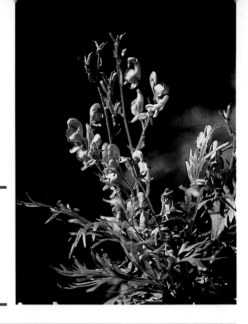

## High temperature
**with sudden onset after exposure to dry cold**

## Acute anxiety
## Hypertension
## Neuralgia

---

### Febrile disorders:
**High temperature** with sudden onset after exposure to dry cold. Dry warm skin; intense thirst; anxious agitation; dry cough.
Hoarseness, croupy cough.
**Otitis** with unbearable pain.
**Heat stroke - sunstroke.**

### Neurological disorders:
Intense **neuralgia** with tingling and numbness, in particular of the trigeminal nerve.

**General excitation** with fear of death.

### Cardiovascular disorders:
Bouts of **hypertension** with tachycardia and palpitations.
Angina pectoris.
Hemorrhages of bright red blood.

### Other disorders:
Amenorrhea, secondary to cold or to a fright.

---

**Aggravation:**
– from dry cold,
– around midnight.

**Improvement:**
– with the onset of sweating (in febrile conditions).

# ACTÆA SPICATA

Baneberry
Ranunculaceae

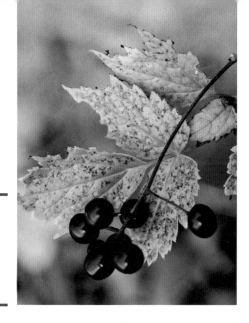

**Rheumatism of the proximal interphalangeal joints**

Deforming rheumatism of the wrists and fingers.

Rheumatoid polyarthritis.

Aggravation:   – from movement,
              – from damp cold.

# AGARICUS MUSCARIUS

Fly agaric
Agaricaceae

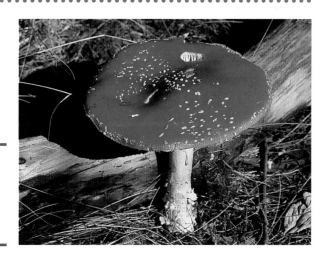

**Spasms**
**Facial tics**
**Chilblains**

**Spasms and contractions** of the limbs and the body. Senile tremor. Facial tics, choreic movements.

Very painful chilblains, with stinging and burning (as if pierced by needles).
**Cyanosis and tumefaction of the hands,** feet, nose, ears.

# ALLIUM CEPA

Onion
Liliaceae

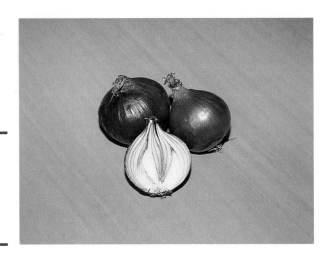

## Acute rhinitis
## Neuralgia

**Rhinitis :**
**Common coryza,** rhinitis (seasonal or otherwise), starting with frequent sneezing and followed by a discharge irritating the nostrils and the upper lip.

**Non-irritant ocular discharge** and painful spasmodic cough, with a rasping or tearing sensation.

**Neuralgia and neuritis:**
Neuritis of amputation stumps.

Aggravation:
– from heat,
– from seasonal allergens.

Improvement:
– in a cool environment.

# ALOE SOCOTRINA

Aloes
Liliaceae

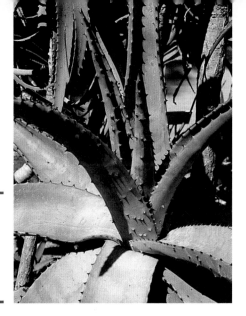

**Diarrhea**
**Hemorrhoids**

**Urgent spurting diarrhea** on waking and immediately after eating or drinking. Abundant gas. Involuntary emission of feces.

Burning **hemorrhoids** "like a bunch of grapes", bluish, oozing, improved by a cold bath.

Aggravation:
– after eating or drinking,
– from beer,
– from heat.

Improvement:
– with cold (local applications on hemorrhoids).

# ALUMINA

Aluminum oxide
Alumina

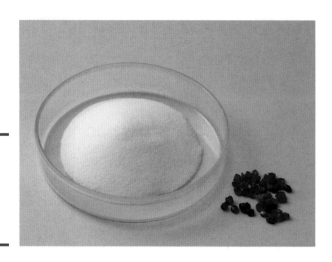

**Constipation**
**Premature ageing**

Constipation from rectal inertia; the stools, even when soft, are only expelled after great effort.

**Dehydration of the skin,** wrinkled, withered aspect.

Disturbances of memory and ideation.
The patient walks slowly, with small steps, trembling and lacking coordination.

Aggravation:
– from cold,
– in the morning on waking.

Improvement:
– in the open air.

# AMMONIUM MURIATICUM

Ammonium chloride

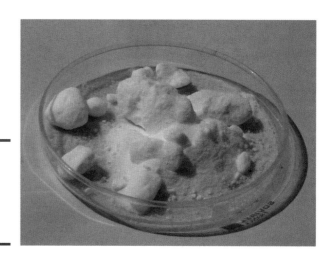

## Rhinitis
## Constipation
## Sciatica

**Rhinitis with clear irritant nasal discharge,** but with the sensation of a blocked nose; total loss of smell.

**Stubborn constipation with much gas.** The stools are hard and crumble into small pieces around the anus.

**Sciatica:** pains aggravated in a sitting position.

Aggravation:
– from cold,
– in a sitting position.

Improvement:
– when walking,
– in a lying position
   (for the pains).

# ANAGALLIS ARVENSIS

Scarlet pimpernel
Primulaceae

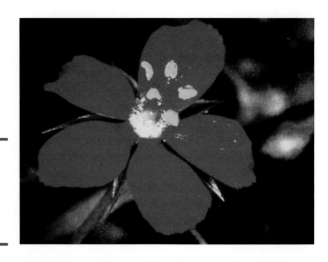

## Vesicles
## Dyshidrosis

Erythematous and vesicular erup-**tions** with violent pruritus in the palms of the hands and soles of the feet.

Palmar and plantar dyshidrosis.

# ANTIMONIUM CRUDUM

Antimony trisulfide

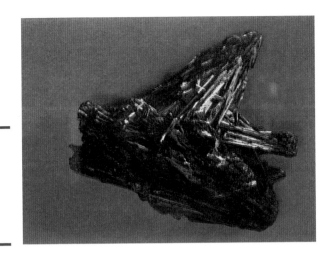

**Overeating
Dermatosis**

**Dyspepsia after overeating:**
Tongue covered with a thick whitish coating on the whole surface.
**Belching with the taste of the ingested food.**
Half-liquid, half-solid diarrhea.
Craving for cured meat products and acidic food or drinks, despite intolerance of them.
Compensatory **overeating:** the medicine is used to moderate the appetite in 30C, 5 pellets, 3 or 4 times a day.

**Dermatosis:**
**Impetigo** on the face around the mouth.
Hard horny **warts,** particularly **plantar.**
Fissures related to hyperkeratosis (heels).

**Aggravation:**
− from overeating,
− from cold baths,
− from radiating heat,
− from vinegary foods.

**Improvement:**
− with warm applications.

# ANTIMONIUM TARTARICUM

Antimony potassium
tartrate
Tartar emetic

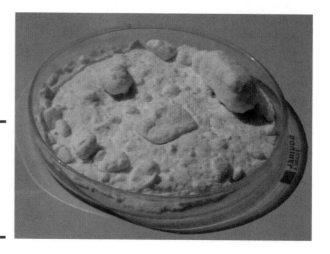

**Dyspnea
Abundant mucus
Difficult
expectoration
Marked pallor**

Intense dyspnea in young children and elderly patients; acute or chronic bronchitis.
Chronic respiratory failure, wheezing, chapped lips, accumulation of mucus in the bronchi.

Thick expectoration, difficult to loosen.

Drowsiness, pallor.

Aggravation:
– from heat,
– in a lying position.

Improvement:
– from expectoration,
– in a sitting position.

Low dilutions increase secretions (and help difficult expectoration); high dilutions dry them up.

# APIS MELLIFICA

Honeybee
Apidae

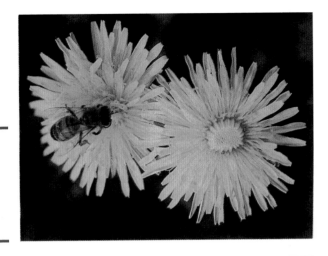

**All types of acute or chronic edema**

Pinkish-red **edema**, with rapid onset, stinging, burning, **relieved by applying cold water;** edema may be local (insect bites or stings) or general. Sunburn; urticaria; first-degree burns. Chilblains with burning pain, as from red-hot needles.

Sudden hydrarthrosis of the knee. Rheumatic pains with swollen red joints.
**Sore throat with edema of the uvula, stinging pains.**
Edematous acute nephritis.
Temperature without thirst.

Eye: pinkish edema, stinging pains, styes, chalazia.

Aggravation:
— from topical or ambient warmth,
— from touch.

Improvement:
— with cold.

# ARGENTUM NITRICUM

Silver nitrate

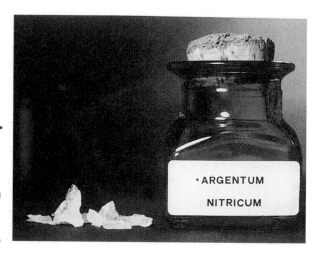

**Anxiety**
**Vertigo**
**Nervous anticipation**
**Ulcerations**

**Anxiety:**
Nervous anticipation or "stage fright" (with nervous diarrhea), **with a hurried feeling, fear of non-achievement.**
Trembling, coordination problems.

Vertigo from heights or when closing the eyes.

**Ulcerations:**
Gastric ulcer.
**Pharyngitis,** laryngitis with pain as from a splinter in the affected mucosa.

Aggravation:
− from sweets and candies,
− when closing the eyes,
− from ambient warmth.

Improvement:
− with cold.

# ARNICA MONTANA

Leopard's bane
Compositae

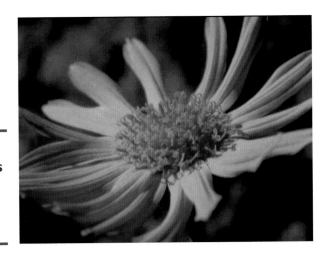

**All types of traumas**
**Overexertion**
**Capillary fragility**

### Traumas:
All shocks, falls, accidents, wounds, surgery, including preventive treatment (also dental surgery).

### Overexertion:
Due to overwork or excessive physical training, with **sensations of contusion, bruising, or aching** (the bed feels too hard).

Straining of the vocal cords (singers, orators).

Cardiovascular strain: **athletic heart;** bouts of hypertension; the head is warm, congested, the body is cold.

### Capillary fragility:
Painful breakage of small peripheral vessels, followed by **hematoma.**
**Epistaxis.**
Nephritis **with hematuria.**
**Painful varicose veins,** sensation of bruising.
Bouts of hemorrhoids.
Bluish or violaceous chilblains.
Fever with hemorrhagic phenomena.

All types of hemorrhage. Childbirth: before, during, and after delivery.

### Aggravation:
— from the slightest touch,
— from jolts,
— from damp cold.

### Improvement:
— with rest,
— in a lying position, with the head low.

# ARSENICUM ALBUM

Arsenic trioxide

---

**Anxiety**
**Burning pain relieved**
**by warmth**
**Weakened general**
**condition**

---

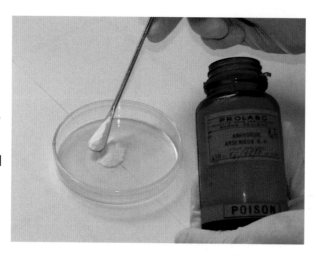

**ENT disorders:**
**Dyspnea from exertion** or in a lying position; asthma attack; **aggravation around 1 a.m.** with extreme chilliness despite a need for fresh air.
Coryza: very irritant and burning discharge. Improvement with warmth.
**Otitis:** burning pains.

**Digestive disorders:**
**Acute gastroenteritis** with burning, nauseous, brownish diarrhea, related to food poisoning.

Aversion for meat, intolerance of fruit, icy drinks and ice-creams; desire for warm drinks.

**Cutaneous disorders:**
**Urticaria, herpes zoster, eczema** with fine desquamation, like rice powder or flakes of bran, improved by warm applications.
**Chilblains** with intense burning.
Eye: burning excoriated eyelid.

Burning neuralgia, improved by warmth.

Aggravation:
– between 1 and 3 a.m.,
– from cold,
– from fruit.

Improvement:
– with warmth and warm applications,
– by changing position.

# ARUM TRIPHYLLUM

Indian turnip
Araceae

---

## Rhinopharyngeal inflammation

---

**Acute rhinopharyngitis,** bright red mucosa of the nose and throat, with burning irritation, stinging, excoriation.

**Very painful laryngitis** of singers and orators. Bitonal hoarse voice, hoarseness with constantly changing tone of voice.
Seasonal laryngitis.

**Lips:** sensation of burning with excoriation that the patient picks at; bleeding.

**Aggravation:**
– from heat.

# ASAFŒTIDA

Devil's dung
Umbelliferae

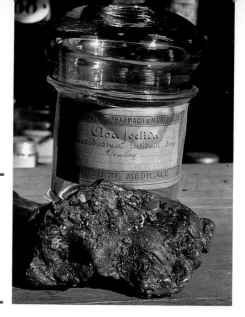

## Spasms

| | |
|---|---|
| **Esophageal spasms** which make swallowing difficult and noisy. Impression of a lump in the larynx rising from below. | **Gastric tympanites.** Aerophagia. Difficult and noisy belching which smells of garlic. |

Aggravation:
– from the slightest touch,
– at night.

Improvement:
– in the open air.

# BADIAGA

Fresh water sponge
Spongillidae

## Spasmodic coryza

| | |
|---|---|
| Profuse watery coryza with **sneezing**. | **Pertussoid cough** with discharge of thready mucus. |

Aggravation:
– from cold.

Improvement:
– with warmth.

# BELLADONNA

Deadly nightshade
Solanaceae

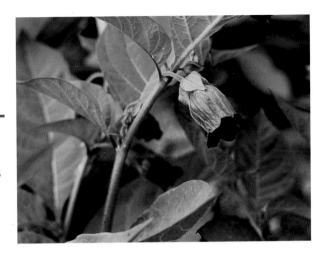

## Temperature
## Dryness of the mucous membranes
## Congestion
## Spasms

tumor- rubor - dolor - calor

**Temperature:**
Sudden and high onset (102.2°F-103.1°F) with a warm red face and profuse sweating. In case of **febrile convulsions,** give **Belladonna** in 30C while waiting for the doctor.

**Intense dryness of the mucous membranes:**
Pharyngitis, rhinopharyngitis, hoarseness, sore throat compelling the patient to swallow very often.
**Tracheitis with dry and painful cough.**
Congestive otitis media with a throbbing pain.

**Congestion:**
**Pulsatile headache,** hot flushes, sunstroke, sunburns, first-degree burns.
Mammary congestion during the breast-feeding period.
**Bouts of hypertension.**
Beginning of dental abscess.
Red eye, sensitive to light (styes, chalazia).

**Spasms:**
Hepatic or renal colic.
**Hiccup.**

**Aggravation:**
– from bright light,
– from noise,
– from touch.

**Improvement:**
– with rest.

# BERBERIS VULGARIS

Barberry
Berberidaceae

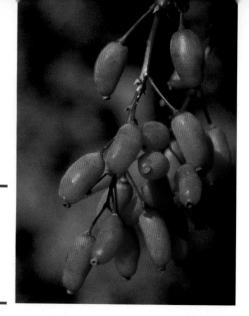

**Kidneys**
**Liver**
**Gallbladder**
**Skin**
**Rheumatism**

### Kidneys:
**Urinary lithiasis;** urine output is variable and insufficient; renal pains mainly on the left, sensation of bruising.

### Liver - Gallbladder:
**Hepatic colic** with pains which radiate, disorders of the hepatovesicular functions with nausea, postprandial drowsiness, discolored stools.

### Skin:
**Dermatosis with a circular shape,** pruriginous, with desquamation in thin flakes; circinate herpes.

### Rheumatism:
Gout and articular manifestations in patients suffering from hyperuricemia.
Lumbar and lumbosacral pains.

Aggravation:
– from the slightest jolt.

Improvement:
– with profuse urine output.

# BORAX

Sodium borate

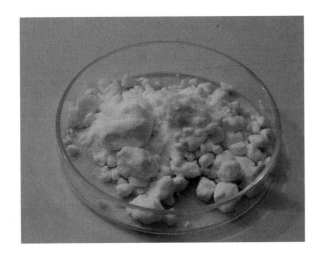

**Aphthae**
**Herpes**
**Fear of downward movement**
**Leukorrhea**

**Canker sores:**
**Oral aphthosis,** often in infants, which prevents them from sucking. In adults: vesicles which are very painful on contact with acidic or salty foods.

**Herpes:**
**Genital** or perioral concomitant with the aphthae.

**Motion sickness:**
From fear of downward movement (planes).

**Leukorrhea:**
**Whitish** and giving the impression of running like warm water, like raw egg white.

Aggravation:
– from downward movement.

# BRYONIA ALBA

White bryony
Cucurbitaceae

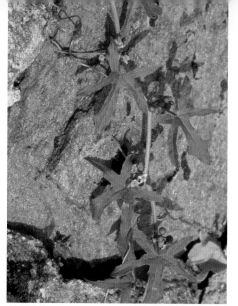

**Inflammation**
**Dryness of mucous membranes**
**Exudation of serous membranes**
**Pains in localized points**

**Inflammation:**
**Fever with progressive onset,** with thirst for large quantities of cold water. The person seeks to remain immobile, lying on the painful side. Sunstroke, heat stroke.

**Dryness of mucous membranes:**
**Dry cough,** painful, tracheitis or bronchitis; intense thirst.
Constipation with dry stools, "as if burnt".

**Exudation of serous membranes:**
**Pleuritis.**
Hydrarthrosis, acute rheumatoid arthritis.

**Pains in localized points:**
Headache with progressive onset, relieved by a tight head-band.
Painful point in the thorax, relieved by strong pressure.
Painful point in the right ovary.
Painful points in the breasts; mastitis, mammary dystrophy.

Aggravation:
– from movement,
– from the slightest touch,
– from heat (except for local pains),
– from meals,
– at around 9 p.m.

Improvement:
– with rest,
– with strong pressure or when lying on the painful side,
– with cold,
– with sweating.

# CALCAREA CARBONICA OSTREARUM

Oyster shell

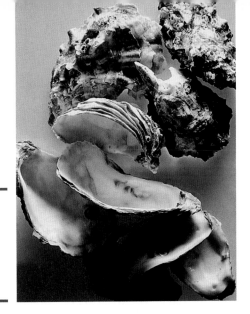

**ENT disorders**
**Cutaneous disorders**
**Nutritional disorders**

**Infants:**
**Infants given too much milk,** or intolerant of milk; vomiting.
Milk crusts - Eczema.
**Wide fontanelle** which is slow to close.
Tendency to perspiration of the head.
**Diaper rash.**

**Children:**
**Recurrent ENT complaints.**
**Slowness,** disinclination for intellectual work.
Late puberty in girls.

**Adults:**
**Nutritional disorders due to ove-reating,** obesity, diabetes, gout, eczema, migraines.
Tendency to polyps.
For young mothers, excessive milk secretion.

Aggravation:
– from damp cold,
– from physical or intellectual effort,
– from milk and dairy products.

Improvement:
– with dry weather.

# CALCAREA FLUORICA

Calcium fluoride

## Asymmetry
## Hyperlaxity

**Asymmetry:**
**Osseous dystrophy,** upper prognathism, markedly ogival roof of the mouth, irregularly disposed teeth.
**Tendency to scoliosis.**
Tendency to osteoporosis.

**Hyperlaxity:**
**Sprains,** recurrent lumbago.
Voluminous varicose veins.
**Visceral ptosis.**

Aggravation:
– from humidity,
– from rest,
– when starting to move.

Improvement:
– with movement,
- with warmth and warm
  applications.

# CALCAREA SULPHURICA

Calcium sulfate

## Prolonged painless suppuration

**Suppuration of cutaneous lesions:**
Thick yellow pus.
No pain, no inflammatory signs.

Helps to drain pus after excision of a felon.

# CALENDULA OFFICINALIS

Garden marigold
Compositae

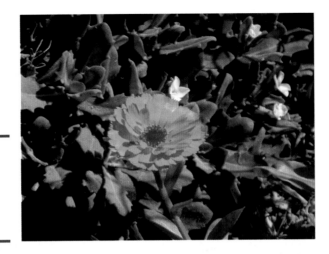

**Wounds and infection**

Used externally as a local antiseptic on the skin and mucous membranes.

Used internally as a hemostatic, antiseptic, antalgic (varicose ulcers).

# CANTHARIS

Spanish fly
Meloideae

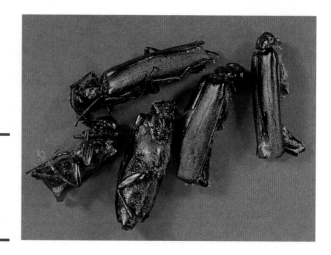

**Vesicles**
**Burns**
**Cystitis**

### Vesicular eruptions:
**Bullous**, burning; herpes, zoster, eczema, pemphigus, burning pruritus.

### Second-degree burns with phlyctena:
From scalding.
From the sun (sunburns, photodermatosis).

### Acute cystitis:
With burning pains before, during, and after each micturition.
Nephritis with hematuria, with unbearable pains.

### Others:
Canker sores and necrotic ulcerating pharyngitis with intense burning.
Gastritis with burning pyrosis.
Acute keratoconjunctivitis.

Aggravation:
– when urinating.

Improvement:
– with warmth,
– when lying.

# CAPSICUM ANNUUM

Red pepper
Solanaceae

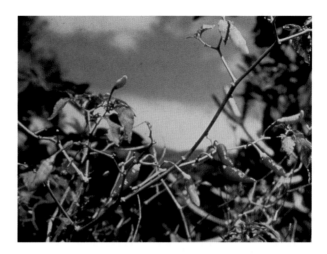

## Inflammation from the mouth to the rectum
with sensation of intense burning "as if pepper had been poured onto it"

Glossitis, stomatitis, pharyngitis. Pyrosis, burning hemorrhoids.

Acute congestive otitis; stabbing earache.
Mastoiditis.

Aggravation:
– from cold,
– from spicy food.

# CARBO VEGETABILIS

Officinal vegetable charcoal
Wood charcoal

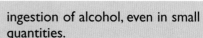

## Tympanites
## Cyanosis

**Gastric and intestinal tympanites (above the navel):**
Aggravated in a lying position, from intolerance to alcohol and fatty food, improved by belching.

**Cyanosis:**
Congestive flushes and erythrocyanosis of the face after ingestion of alcohol, even in small quantities.
Atonic ulcers.
Raynaud's syndrome.
Chilblains.
Acute or chronic **respiratory failure** in elderly patients.
Whooping cough.

Aggravation:
– from alcohol,
– from fatty food.

Improvement:
– with belching,
– on being fanned.

# CASTOR EQUI

Horse chestnut (primitive thumbnail of the horse)

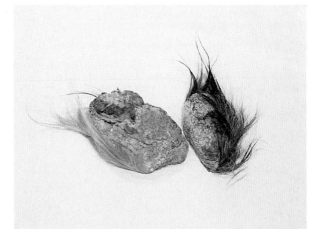

Cracks of the nipples during the breast-feeding period.

Bedsores.

# CAULOPHYLLUM

Blue cohosh
Berberidaceae

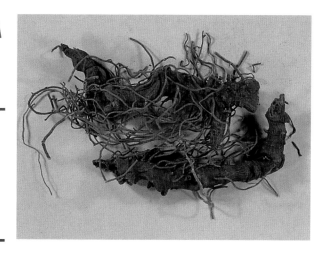

**Menstrual pains
Delivery pains
Pains of the small
joints**

**Early menses,** painful, with cramps and spasms, scanty.

**Delivery:** interruption of labor with rigidity of the cervix, atonia of the uterus, and interrupted dilation.

Pains of the small interphalangeal joints.

# CAUSTICUM

Complex chemical substance obtained by distillation of a mixture of freshly slaked lime and potassium bisulfate

**Burning of the mucous membranes**
**Paralysis**
**Stiffness**
**Warts**

**Burning of the mucous membranes:**
Painful cough, burning in the trachea, radiating pain in the hips.

**Paralysis:**
**With premature atrophy and stiffness.**
Facial paralysis, paralysis of the vocal cords with constant hoarseness, burning and rasping sensation in the larynx. Difficulty swallowing. Constipation.

Urinary incontinence from effort, when coughing.

**Stiffness:**
Painful stiffness, **tendinitis, writers' cramp,** coxarthrosis. Improvement in rainy weather and with warmth.

**Warts:**
**Under the nails or on the face.**

Senile pruritus improved by scratching.
Painful or pruriginous keloid scars.

Aggravation:
– from dry cold,
– around 3 a.m. and in the evening.

Improvement:
– with warmth,
– in damp weather.

# CHAMOMILLA

German chamomile
Compositae

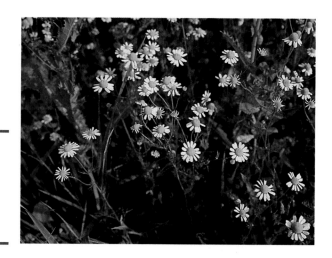

**Problems
with teething
Intolerance to pain**

**Problems with teething:**
Pain which makes the infant grumpy, irascible, capricious.
**Fever with a single red and warm cheek.**

**Intolerance to pain in cases of:**
Dental neuralgia, sciatica.
Hepatic and renal colic.

Otitis with unbearable pain.
Pain provoking anger in persons who are usually calm.

Aggravation:
— from anger,
— from upsets,
— from coffee and stimulants,
— in the evening before midnight.

Improvement:
— with passive movement (being rocked for children, or when riding in a car or train).

# CHEIRANTHUS CHEIRI

Wallflower
Cruciferae

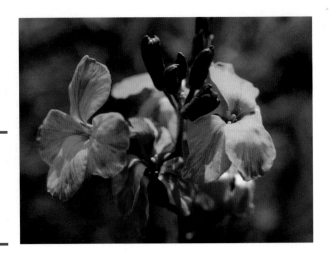

**Trismus associated
with problems
caused by wisdom
teeth**

# CHELIDONIUM MAJUS

Greater celandine
Papaveraceae

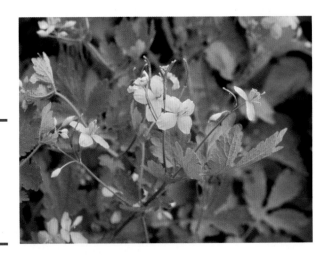

**Hepatobiliary
syndrome
Fixed pain at the
lower angle of the
right scapula**

Constipation with discolored stools.     Postprandial drowsiness.

Local applications of mother tincture as a complement in the treatment of warts.

**Aggravation:**
– from heat,
– at 4 a.m. and 4 p.m.

**Improvement:**
– after having ingested warm foods
  or drinks,
– with pressure.

# CIMICIFUGA RACEMOSA or ACTAEA RACEMOSA

Black cohosh
Ranunculaceae

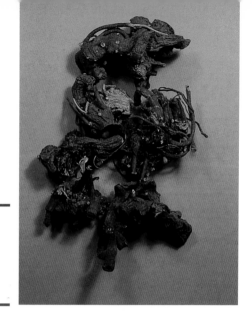

## Gynecological and neuromuscular disorders

**Gynecological disorders:**
**Painful ovulation,** with hemorrhaging.
**Cramping menstrual pain,** proportional to the menstrual flow, compelling the patient to bend double.
Irregular, spasmodic, painful labor (childbirth) .
"**Cimicifuga racemosa** is the younger woman's **Lachesis**."

**Neuromuscular disorders:**
**Backache,** particularly involving the first four dorsal vertebrae. Cervical pain.
Torticollis improved by holding the head back.
**Tendinitis.**

Aggravation:
– during menses,
– from cold.

Improvement:
– with warmth.

# CINA

Santonica
Compositae

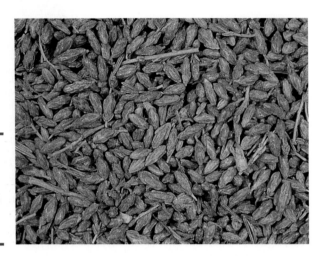

**Disorders related to
intestinal parasitosis**

Periumbilical colic, better when lying prone.
Grinding of teeth.
Spasmodic cough, often at night.

Nasal and anal pruritus.
Pale complexion of the face and bluish rings around the eyes.
Enuresis.

Aggravation:
— at night,
— with the new moon and the full moon,
— from attention.

Improvement:
— when lying prone.

# CINCHONA OFFICINALIS

Red cinchona
Rubiaceae

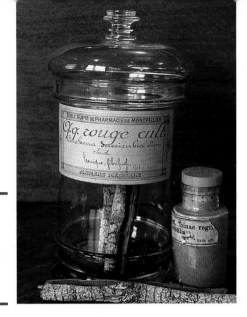

## General weakness
following profuse loss of organic liquid or prolonged fevers

### Loss of organic fluid:
Hemorrhages: epistaxis, menometrorrhagia of dark blood with pallor of the face.
As repeated hemorrhages lead to hypochromic and sideropenic anemia, **Cinchona officinalis** can be given preventively before surgery.
Painless but exhausting diarrhea, with profuse foul-smelling gas, after having eaten fruit or drunk milk. Most often, marked abdominal tympanites.

### Fevers:
Influenzal or pseudo-influenzal syndromes.
Periodic fevers (malaria) in precise successive phases; shivering, heat, sweating.

### Aggravation:
– from loss of liquid,
– from slight touch,
– from drafts.

### Improvement:
– with warmth,
– with strong pressure.

# COCCULUS INDICUS

Fish berry
Menispermaceae

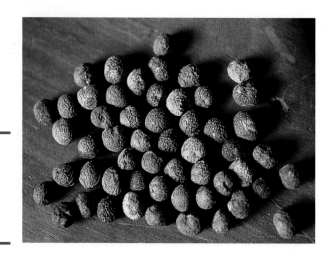

## Motion sickness

**Motion sickness with vertigo, nausea,** vomiting, aggravated by eating, not relieved by fresh air.

Vomiting of pregnancy.
Spasmodic pains during menses, with hemorrhage of dark blood, with nausea, vertigo, insomnia.

**Aggravation:**
- from staying up late,
- from overwork,
- from passive movement (car, train, boat).

**Improvement:**
- with warmth,
- in a confined environment.

# COCCUS CACTI

Cochineal
Coccidae

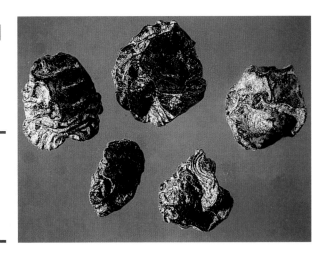

**Whooping cough
Fitful cough**

**Whooping cough:**
Fully-declared phase.

**Fitful cough:**
**Due to laryngeal tickling** with marked catarrh and discharge of profuse thready mucus.

Aggravation:
– in a warm room,
– in the morning.

Improvement:
– in a cold room,
– with cold drinks.

# COLOCYNTHIS

Bitter apple
Cucurbitaceae

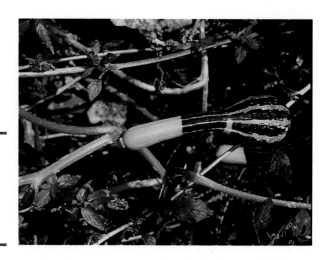

**Pains compelling
the person to bend
double**

Troubles digestifs :
**Hepatic colic,** violent cramping
pains.
Spasmodic colonopathy.
Painful **diarrhea,** visceral cramping
pains, relieved by bending double.
**Digestion is blocked by anger.**

Urinary disorders:
Renal colic.

Genital disorders:
Cramping pains.

Neuralgic disorders:
Facial neuralgia, trigeminal nerve.
Sciatic neuralgia.

Aggravation:
– from anger.

Improvement:
– with pressure.

# CONDURANGO

Eagle vine
Asclepiadaceae

---

**Perlèche**
**Gastric ulcers**
**Anal fissures**

---

Ulcerated fissures at the corner of the mouth and in the anus.

Esophageal and gastric pains with burning.

# CORALLIUM RUBRUM

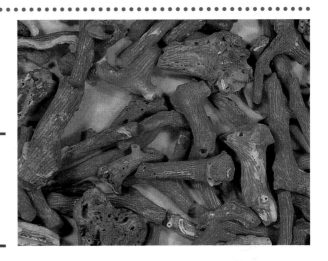

Red coral
Coralliidae

---

**Pertussoid cough**

---

**Explosive cough** in violent fits, with vomiting of thick thready mucus, leaving the person exhausted. The face flushes scarlet during the coughing fit, which is triggered by cold air or eating.

Aggravation:
– from exposure to cool air,
– at night.

Improvement:
– with warmth.

# CUPRUM METALLICUM

Metallic copper

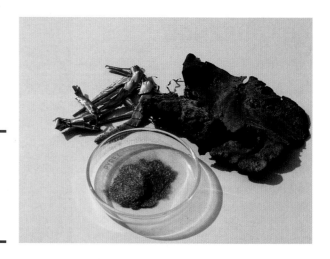

**Cramps**
**Spasms**
**Diarrhea**

## On the striated muscles:
**Cramps** of the calves and toes occuring at night (as a preventive measure, give 5 pellets of **Cuprum metallicum** in 6C before going to bed, to be repeated in case of cramps).
Writers' cramp.
Painful facial tics
**Hiccup** relieved by drinking cold water.

## On the smooth muscles:
Very violent, spasmodic **colic.**
**Whooping cough, spasmodic cough** with cyanosis.

**Aggravation:**
– from cold,
– at night.

**Improvement:**
– by drinking cold water.

# DIOSCOREA VILLOSA

Wild yam
Dioscoreaceae

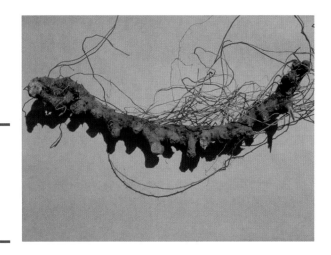

## Visceral pains

**or neuralgia relieved by hyperextension**

**Cramping pains,** sudden, acute, paroxysmal, recurring at regular intervals, relieved by hyperextension, aggravated by flexion.

Gastric pains, intestinal or uterine. Back pains, lumbosacral pains.

Aggravation:
– from flexion.

Improvement:
– with extension.

# DROSERA ROTUNDIFOLIA

Sundew
Droseraceae

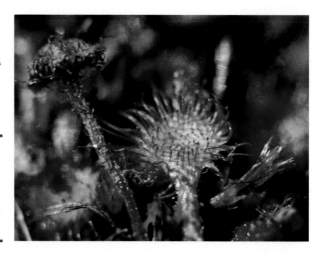

**Fitful cough**
**Adenopathy**

**Coughing fits** in the evening after midnight or immediately after going to bed; suffocating spasmodic cough; costal or abdominal pains which compel the patient to grip his belly, accompanied by vomiting of thready mucus; sensation of laryngeal tickling "as with a feather".

General asthenia, **cervical and tracheobronchial adenopathy** which trigger coughing by compression.

Aggravation:
– at night after midnight,
– in a lying position,
– from warmth in bed.

Improvement:
– with movement,
– with local pressure (by pressing the ribcage).

# DULCAMARA

Bittersweet
Solanaceae

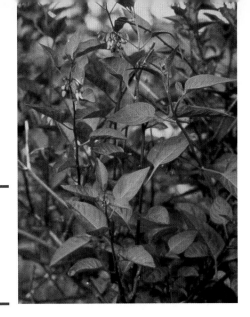

**Disorders triggered
by damp cold**
(fog)

**Respiratory disorders:**
**Rhinopharyngitis,** bronchitis, asthma
after exposure to damp cold.

**Cutaneous disorders:**
Urticaria from cold.
Translucent flat warts.

**Digestive disorders:**
Diarrhea after a chill.

**Rheumatic pain** aggravated by
humidity.

Aggravation :
— from damp cold, rain, fog;
— at night.

Improvement:
— in warm dry weather.

# EUPATORIUM PERFOLIATUM

Boneset
Compositae

---

**Influenzal aches and pains**
**Pain of the eyeballs**

---

Influenza and influenzal syndromes with tenderness of the eyeballs, muscular aching, sensation that the bones are broken, intense thirst for cold water.

**Aggravation:**
– from pressure on the eyeballs.

# EUPHRASIA OFFICINALIS

Eyebright
Scrophulariaceae

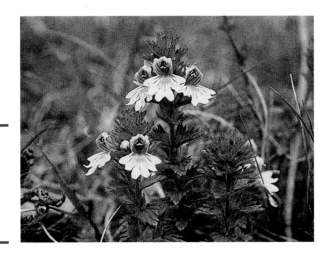

## Irritant lacrimation

Inflammation of the nasal and ocular mucous membranes with lacrimation irritating the conjunctiva, the eyelids, the cornea; sensation of sand in the eyes, with a clear nasal discharge, profuse but not irritant.

**Aggravation:**
– from heat,
– from light,
– from wind.

**Improvement:**
– in the dark.

# FERRUM PHOSPHORICUM

Ferrosoferric phosphate

---

## Mild inflammation
## Minor hemorrhages

---

Eruptive diseases with progressive onset, with slight fever, alternating pallor and redness of the face, moist skin.
**Moderate fever** (100.4°F-101.3°F).
Acute congestive otitis.
Rhinopharyngitis with epistaxis.

**Dry cough,** blood-streaked expectoration.

Infantile diarrhea streaked with blood.

Aggravation:
– in a lying position,
– from cold air.

Improvement:
– with topical cold.

# GALPHIMIA GLAUCA

Shower of Gold
Malpighiaceae

---

**Hay fever**

---

**Nose and eye discharge** often accompagnied by edema of the eyelids and sneezing.

# GELSEMIUM SEMPERVIRENS

Yellow jasmine
Loganiaceae

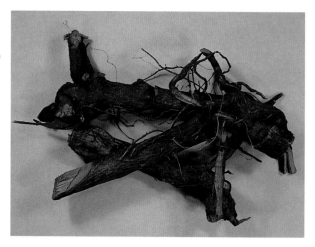

**Influenza**
**Nervous**
**apprehension**
**Paralysis**

## Influenza:

Slight fever with progressive onset, influenzal syndrome with general weakness, drowsiness, **prostration**, crimson face, absence of thirst, and generalized aches and pains.
Occipital headache with diplopia.
Coryza with acrid and excoriating discharge.

## Nervous apprehension:

**Gelsemium sempervirens** is the major medicine for nervous apprehension with loss of confidence, loss of memory, trembling, emotional diarrhea.
Insomnia due to anticipation anxiety.
Fear of going to the dentist.
Anxiety before surgery.

Post-herpetic facial paralysis.
Painful and ineffective labor during delivery.

## Aggravation:
– from hot weather,
– from emotions.

## Improvement:
– with fresh air,
– with movement,
– with profuse micturition.

# GLONOINUM

Nitroglycerin
Trinitrin

---

## Cerebral congestion

---

**Sudden congestive headache** with intense and visible throbbing of the carotid artery, relieved by pressing the head between the hands and by cold applications.

After a sunstroke or in hypertensive patients.

**Tachycardia,** tachyarrhythmia. Congestive hypertension.

**Hot flushes of the menopause.**

Aggravation:
– from radiating heat,
– from jolts,
– from noise.

Improvement:
– in the open air,
– when pressing the head between the hands.

# GRAPHITES

Plumbago
Black lead

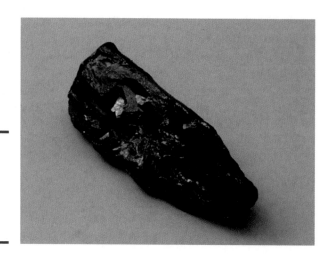

**Eczema
Constipation
Chilliness**

Cutaneous disorders:
**Eczematous eruptions,** yellowish oozing vesicles, with pruritus and burning, becoming covered with small scabs.
**Fissures** of the nipples, tips of the fingers. Keloid scars (as soon as they appear).
Painful warts around the nails.

Digestive disorders:
**Atonic chronic constipation,** without urge, with voluminous stools held together by mucus.
**Bloatedness** and intolerance to tight clothes.
Hemorrhoids with painful and oozing fissures.

Aggravation:
– from cold,
– from warmth in bed,
– during menses.

Improvement:
– with movement in the open air,
– when eating.

# HEKLA LAVA

Lava from Mount Hekla

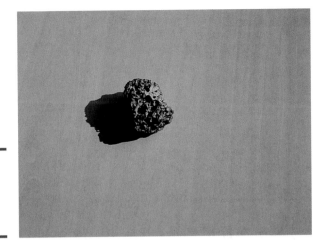

**Exostosis**

Neoformative **bony outgrowths**, whatever their causes. Calcaneus spine.

Inflammation of the maxilla, osteitis, osteoarthritis, hallux valgus. Post-traumatic reactions affecting the periosteum.

# HEPAR SULPHURIS CALCAREUM

Crude calcium sulfide

According to Hahnemann, it is a mixture of equal parts of purified flowers of sulfur and of powdered oyster shells. The mode of preparation is described in the Homeopathic Pharmacopeia of the United States HPUS.

## Inflammation
## Suppuration

**Inflammation:**
**Acute laryngitis** with splintering pain, **hoarse barking cough,** hypersensitivity to pain.
Tracheobronchitis.

**Suppuration:**
"**Any small wound suppurates.**"
Purulent conjunctivitis, purulent coryza, purulent sinusitis, dental abscess.
These discharges always smell foul.

**Aggravation:**
— from cold and drafts;
— from the slightest touch.

**Improvement:**
— with warmth.

Low dilutions cause pus to gather.
High dilutions dry up pus.
Beware of using **Hepar sulphuris calcareum** in case of closed cavities where the pus cannot drain.

# HYDRASTIS CANADENSIS

Goldenseal
Ranunculaceae

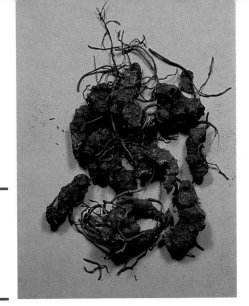

## Hepatovesicular and ENT syndromes

**Disorders of the mucous membranes:**
Rhinitis, sinusitis with secretions that are thick, yellowish, viscous, and posterior nasal flow, forming plugs.
Chronic bronchitis of smokers, of elderly patients.
Yellow leukorrhea with pruritus.
Chronic urethritis.

**Digestive disorders:**
Anorexia with sensation of emptiness in the pit of the stomach and intense weakness not improved when eating.
Aphthosis or oral herpes.
Nausea.
Chronic constipation, without urge, after excessive use of laxatives.

Aggravation:
— from cold, in the open air;
— from bread;
— from laxatives.

# HYDROFLUORICUM ACIDUM

Hydrofluoric acid

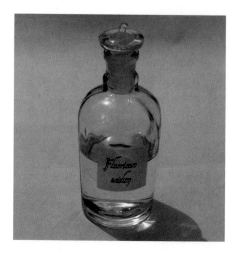

**Demineralization**
**Ulcers**
**Varicose veins**

**Demineralization of the osseous tissue,** osteoporosis, maxillary necrosis, dental fistulae.
Tooth decay of the roots.

**Varicose ulcers** with burning pains, aggravated by heat, varicose veins, varicose eczema with violent pruritus.

Anal pruritus improved by cold applications.

Fissure due to hyperkeratosis of the skin (on the shin).

Aggravation:
– from heat,
– from standing.

Improvement:
– with cold and cold applications.

# HYPERICUM PERFORATUM

St John's wort
Hypericaceae

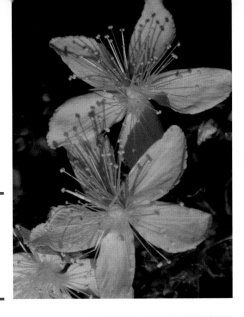

## Pains of the nerve endings

**"The Arnica of the nerves"**

**Traumatism of the nerve endings,** crushing of the extremities, torn-out nails, deep stings or puncture wounds, pains of amputated stumps. These pains are acute, shooting, tearing, unbearable.

**Zoster or post-zoster pains.**
**After a tooth extraction,** as a preventive measure against the risk of alveolitis.
Pains of the coccyx.
Sciatica after surgery.

Aggravation:
– from humidity,
– from cold,
– from jolts.

# IGNATIA AMARA

St Ignatius' bean
Loganiaceae

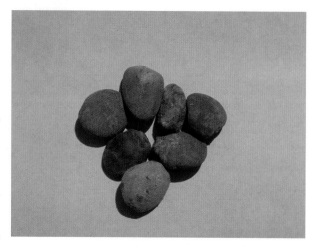

**Hypersensitivity to emotions**
**Paradoxical behavior**

**Depressive disorders:**
Intense asthenia after an emotional blow.
Depression, **silent grief, deep sighs;** the person cries easily but also changes mood rapidly, switches from laughter to tears and vice-versa; quickly consoled by distraction.
**Nervous apprehension with the sensation of a lump in the throat.**

**Spasmodic functional disorders induced by hyperemotivity:**
Digestion is blocked after an upset.
**Emotional tachycardia.**
Spasmodic cough.
Pains localized in points in the appendicular area (without appendicitis) and in the cardiac area (functional pains).
Spasmodic yawning.
Nausea triggered by the slightest odor, improved when eating.

Aggravation:
– from emotions,
– from stimulants,
– from consolation.

Improvement:
– with distraction,
– with strong pressure (on the painful points).

# INFLUENZINUM

Dilution of influenzal vaccine
Nosode

---

**After-effects of flu vaccination,
or flu-like symptoms.**

---

# IPECACUANHA

Ipecac
Rubiaceae

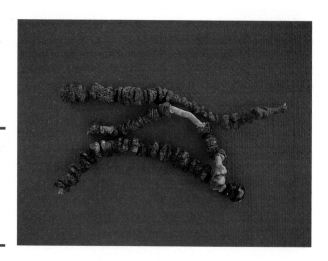

**Reflex nausea
accompanying all
symptoms**

**Digestive disorders:**
**Violent nausea with vomiting** which does not bring relief, hypersalivation. Clear tongue, pale face, bluish rings under the eyes or crimson face and dyspnea.
**Acute diarrhea,** dysenteric, with much mucus, more or less blood-streaked greenish stools, with vomiting, after ingestion of unripe fruit.

**Respiratory disorders:**
**Spasmodic cough** with suffocation, nausea and vomiting, whooping cough and pertussoid cough.
**Hemoptysis** of bright red blood with cough, nausea, vomiting.
Reflex nausea when undergoing dental treatment.

Aggravation:
– from cold,
– from humid heat,
– from movement.

# IRIS VERSICOLOR

Blue flag
Iridaceae

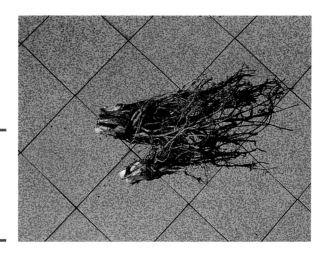

**Burning of the entire digestive tube**
**Ophthalmic migraine**

**Gastroesophageal** burning, burning reflux right up to the mouth.

Recurrent **ophthalmic migraine** (week-end migraine), preceded by visual fogginess.

# KALI BICHROMICUM

Potassium dichromate

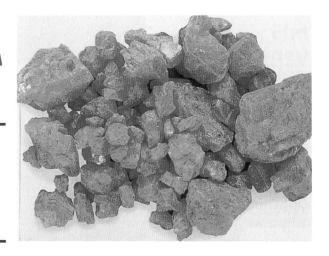

## Mucopurulent secretions Ulcerations

### Digestive disorders:
**Oral aphthosis** (canker sores) with deep ulcerations, as if stamped out with a hole-punch. Ulcerations of the soft palate with edema of the uvula. Round ulcer of the stomach, causing burning, pyrosis.
Intolerance of beer.

### Respiratory disorders:
**Acute or chronic rhinitis, sinusitis** with discharge of thick, greenish-yellow, sticky mucus, forming crusts in the nostrils.

### Cutaneous disorders:
**Varicose ulcers** as if stamped out with a punch-hole.
Dermatosis with scabs and sticky yellow secretion.
Eczema of cement workers.
Pains focused in circumscribed points.

### Aggravation:
– from cold, from cool air;
– when undressing;
– from drinking beer.

### Improvement:
– with warmth.

# KALI BROMATUM

Potassium bromide

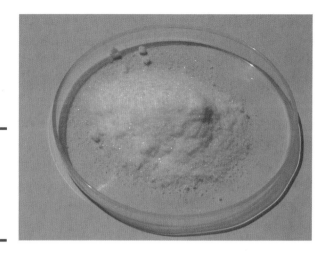

**Instability**
**Acne**
**Pinworms**

Mental disorders:
**Instability with constant agitation of the hands and fingers.**
Memory disturbances.
Intellectual deficiency after over-work.
Difficulty falling asleep and night terrors.

Cutaneous disorders:
**Pustular acne,** with cysts, leaving scars on the face and the upper back.

Pinworms:
**Agitated child, constantly moving hands,** night terrors.

Aggravation:
– with the new moon,
– at night,
– from the slightest intellectual exertion.

Improvement:
– when moving (hands and feet),
– when distracted.

# KALI IODATUM

Potassium iodide

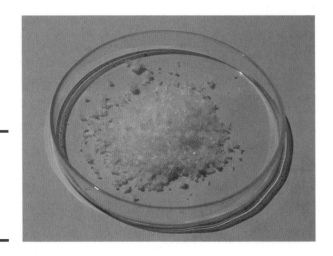

**Rhinitis**
**Sinusitis**
**Rheumatism**

Respiratory disorders:
**Rhinitis with burning watery discharge,** profuse, sneezing and lacrimation. The nose is red, swollen, with a constrictive pain at the root of the nose.
**Acute sinusitis with pains of the frontal sinuses.**
Edema of the uvula, the larynx.

Rheumatic disorders:
**Rheumatism** aggravated at night, by warm humid wind.
Osseous pain at night.
**Articular pain** with a need to move and to be in the open air.
The knees, heels, toes are affected, with **deformities.**

Aggravation:
– at night,
– from heat.

Improvement:
– with fresh air,
– with movement.

# KALI MURIATICUM

Potassium chloride

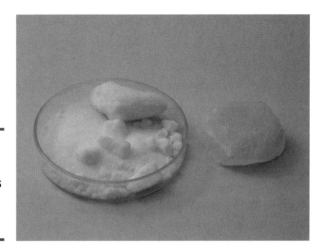

## Thick whitish mucus

**ENT disorders:**
**Tonsillar crypts** with thick whitish caesum, with an unpleasant odor.
**Tubal catarrh** with intermittent deafness, cracking and popping sounds in the ears.

**Digestive disorders:**
**Hepatobiliary dyspepsia** with headache and vomiting of white and thick mucus. Tongue covered with a white coating.

**Cutaneous disorders:**
**Post-inflammatory or chronic edema.** Painful cellulitic edema.
Eruption of vesicles containing a thick white liquid, followed by fine desquamation (zoster, eczema, herpes).

Aggravation:
– from the cold open air,
– from humidity.

Improvement:
– with dry warmth.

# LAC CANINUM

Bitch's milk
Mammals

## Contact hypersensitivity
## of the breasts

symptoms shift from one side to the other

Painful swelling of the breasts before menses, aggravated by touch and jolts, improved during menses. Milk secretion is too profuse after delivery.

All types of pain or inflammation shifting from one side to the other.
Migraines.
Tonsillitis and sore throat.
Ovarialgia.
Rheumatism.

Aggravation:
– from touch, jolts;
– before menses.

Improvement:
– with cold applications
  (rheumatism).

# LACHESIS MUTUS

Bushmaster
Viperidae

**Menopause**
**Alcoholism**
**Sore throat**

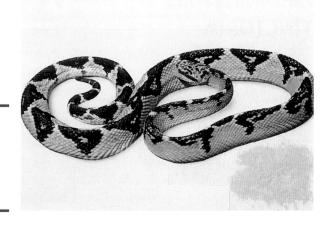

## Disorders of the menopause:
**Menses are diminished or interrupted for several months** with metrorrhagia of blackish blood, hot flushes, spontaneous ecchymoses; throbbing, occipital, left-sided, congestive headache.
High blood pressure.
**Disturbance of mood and behavior,** alternation of excitement and depression.
Jealousy, suspiciousness.
Sensation of constriction, intolerance to collars, scarves, necklaces.

## Disorders of alcoholism:
**Digestive disorders of alcoholics,** with loss of appetite, painful hypertrophic liver.
Bluish-purple hemorrhoids.

## ENT disorders:
**Sore throat shifting from left to right or localized on the left.** The mucous membranes are bluish-purple and it is very difficult for the patient to swallow liquids, especially hot.

## Aggravation:
– from diminution or disappearance of a discharge;
– from touch;
– from all types of heat, the sun;
– on waking.

## Improvement:
– with onset of a natural or pathological discharge;
– in the open air.

# LACHNANTHES TINCTORIA

Red root
Haemodoraceae

---

## Torticollis
## Cervical neuralgia

---

Acute torticollis, mainly on the right, stiffness and contracture of the sternocleidomastoid muscle. All types of cervical pain.

**Aggravation:**
– from rotation of the cervical spine.

# LEDUM PALUSTRE

Wild rosemary
Ericaceae

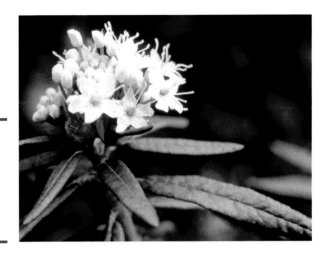

## Traumatic ecchymosis, persistent hematoma
**"black eye"**

Wounds from piercing (nails, thorns) **which do not bleed.**

**Insect bites or stings.** Can be used preventively for people prone to insect bites or stings.

Gout of the large toe. Improvement when walking on a cold floor.

Rheumatism aggravated by heat and in bed.

Aggravation:
– from warmth in bed,
– from movement.

Improvement:
– with cold contact (floor, bath).

# LYCOPODIUM

Club moss
Lycopodiaceae

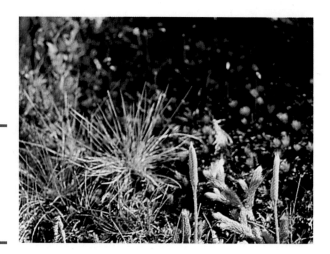

**Hepatic and
digestive disorders
Abdominal
tympanites**

Postprandial drowsiness and malaise.
Intolerance to oysters, garlic, onions.
Marked hunger leading to bad mood, but quickly satiated. Hunger at night.
Pyrosis, burning gastroesophageal reflux.
Distended abdomen, particularly in the lower part.
Varied disorders in patients with hepatic complaints.

Sore throat: right-sided, moving to the left.
Chronic obstruction of the nose.
Impotence, premature ejaculation.
Red sand in the urine.
Irritability.

In infants, digestive problems and anorexia.
In children, cyclic vomiting.

Aggravation:
– from fatty matters,
– from oysters,
– in the late afternoon (5 p.m.).

Improvement:
– with hot drinks,
– in the open air.

# MAGNESIA CARBONICA

Magnesium carbonate

---

**Acidic and flatulent dyspepsia**
**Acute shooting pains**

---

**Digestive disorders:**
**Gastralgia.**
Colic with intestinal pain.
Improvement when bending double, aggravation with dairy products.
Frothy green diarrhea in infants ("frog spawn") caused by milk.
**Tympanites not relieved by passing gas.**

**Neuralgia:**
Improved by walking, strong pressure, hyperflexion.

Sour, acidic sweat.
Blepharitis.
Chronic or recurrent pharyngitis.

**Aggravation:**
– at night,
– from rest.

**Improvement:**
– by bending forward,
– with movement.

# MAGNESIA PHOSPHORICA

Magnesium phosphate

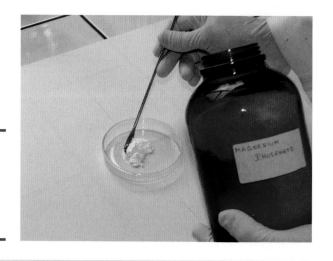

## Spasms
## Cramps
## Neuralgia
**relieved by forced flexion**

**Spasms with a sudden onset and end,** with violent pains making the patient cry out, improved when bending forward, by topical warmth, by strong pressure.
Hepatic, renal, intestinal colic.
Uterine spasms (menses).
Delivery pains.

Writers' cramp, musicians' cramp. Spasmodic hiccup.

**Neuralgia:** facial, with spasms and cramps.
Sciatica improved when flexing the leg onto the pelvis and with warm applications.

Aggravation:
– from cold.

Improvement:
– by forced flexion,
– with warm applications,
– with strong pressure.

# MERCURIUS IODATUS RUBER

Mercuric iodide

# MERCURIUS IODATUS FLAVUS

Mercurous iodide

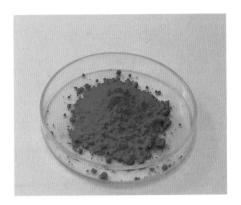

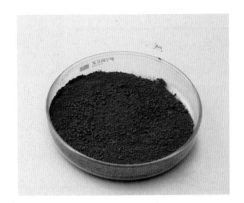

One-sided tonsillitis

on the left for **iodatus ruber (red).**

on the right for **iodatus flavus (yellow).**

# MERCURIUS CORROSIVUS

Mercuric chloride

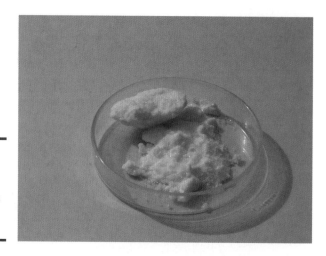

## Ulcerative and hemorrhagic lesions

**Digestive disorders:**
Ulcerative and hemorrhagic gingivostomatitis.
**Intense intestinal pains** with tenesmus, bloody, glairy stools.

**Urogenital disorders:**
**Acute cystitis** with tenesmus and hemorrhaging.

**ENT:**
Pharyngitis and tonsillitis with burning pains, intense pain when swallowing.
Ulcerative and hemorrhagic tonsillitis.
Keratitis.

**Aggravation:**
— from the slightest touch,
— at night.

# MERCURIUS SOLUBILIS

Prepared from mercuric nitrate, nitric acid, and metallic mercury

---

## Mucopurulent secretions:

**"discharges are always foul-smelling"**

---

### ENT disorders:
**Acute or chronic tonsillitis.**
**Coryza with corrosive mucopurulent nasal discharge,** with much sneezing.
Sinusitis with pains.
**Mumps.**
Mucopurulent loose cough.

### Digestive disorders:
Fetid breath.
**Tongue retaining lateral teeth-marks.**

Intense thirst despite hypersalivation.
**Greenish diarrhea,** glairy or blood-streaked.

### Dental problems:
Gingivitis, stomatitis, alveolodental pyorrhea.

Trembling of the extremities, aggravated by emotions and tiredness.
Sweating which does not relieve during febrile episodes.

Aggravation:
– at night,
– from damp cold.

Improvement:
– in a moderately warm and dry atmosphere

**Mercurius vivus** is prepared from metallic mercury. The pathogeneses of **Mercurius vivus** and **Mercurius solubilis** are identical.

# MEZEREUM

Mezereon
Thymelaeaceae

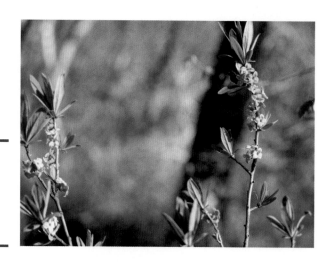

**Cutaneous
eruptions
Neuralgia**

**Cutaneous eruptions:**
**Herpes simplex with vesicles** filled with an opalescent liquid, subsequently covered by a scab with underlying pus.
**Impetigo - herpes zoster.**

**Neuralgia:**
Intercostal, facial, often post-herpetic.
**Osseous pains:** maxillary bone, bones of the face, skull, **long bones.**

**Aggravation:**
– at night from bed warmth,
– from light touch.

**Improvement:**
– with warm applications,
– in the open air.

# MILLEFOLIUM

Yarrow – "Nose-bleed"
Compositae

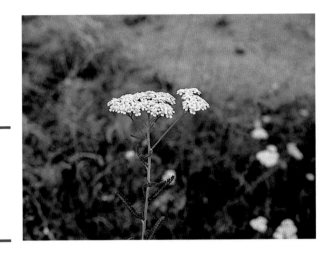

**Hemorrhages**

---

**Spontaneous or traumatic hemorrhages of fluid bright red blood.**
Epistaxis.
Hemorrhages replacing menses.

Prevention of hemorrhaging during dental extraction (with **Phosphorus**).

---

# MONILIA ALBICANS

Candida albicans

**Mycosis**
**Candidiasis**

---

Mainly used in the treatment of **recurrent candidiasis, involving the mouth, skin, or vagina,** or mycosis after treatment with antibiotics.

Give unit-doses in a scale: 9-12-15-30 C.
Repeat the following month if necessary.

# MYRISTICA SEBIFERA

Brazilian ucuba
Myristicaceae

---

**Abscess**
**Felon**

---

Used to accelerate maturation and suppuration of abscesses and felons (with **Hepar sulphuris calcareum**).

Used externally, in ointment or compresses.

· · · · · · · · · · · · · · · · · · · · · · · · · · · · · · · · · · · · · · · · · · · · · · · · · · · ·

# NAPHTHALINUM

Naphthalene

---

**Coryza**

---

**Spasmodic coryza** with irritant nasal and ocular catarrh, much sneezing, pertussoid cough, asthma.

Senile cataract related to diabetes, high blood pressure, albuminuria.

Improvement:
– in the open air for spasmodic
   coryza.

# NATRUM MURIATICUM

Sea salt

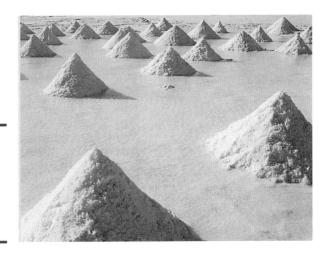

**Nutritional disorders**
**Loss of weight**
**Dehydration**
**Depression**

## Nutritional disorders:
Loss of weight despite a hearty appetite.
Tongue with a "mapped" appearance.
**Intense thirst.**
**Craving for salt or salty food or total rejection of salty food** with stubborn constipation, dry and hard stools.
Physical and intellectual fatigue. Headache.
Convalescence after a severe disease.

## Cutaneous disorders:
Dehydration of the skin with a withered aspect, premature ageing, or oily skin.
Warts in the folds.
Vertical fissure in the middle of the lower lip.
Acne with comedones on the face.
Solar urticaria.
**Herpes simplex.**

## Depression:
Hyperemotivity, depression aggravated by consolation.

Aggravation:
– at the seaside,
– from the sun and heat,
– from grief,
– from consolation.

Improvement:
– in the open air,
– with perspiration.

# NATRUM SULPHURICUM

Sodium sulfate

**Tendency to imbibition
of the tissues
Warts
Chronic mucopurulent
excretions
Depression**

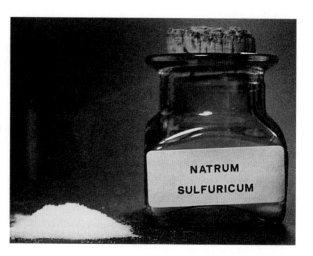

**Water retention -** cellulitis (particularly abdomen and thighs).

**Watery morning diarrhea.**
Flatulence.

**Catarrh of the mucous membranes** with yellow and greenish secretions; all types of bronchopneumopathy aggravated by humidity.

**Coxarthrosis and chronic lumbago** with articular stiffness, improved by movement, aggravated by humidity.

**Desquamative dermatosis** with large fine and transparent scales, with shiny red underlying dermis.
Palmar or plantar dyshidrosis.

Postconcussional syndromes: irritability, depression, stubborn pains.

Aggravation:
– from cold or warm humidity,
– from immobility.

Improvement:
– with dry weather,
– by changing position,
– after profuse stools or by passing wind.

# NITRICUM ACIDUM

Nitric acid

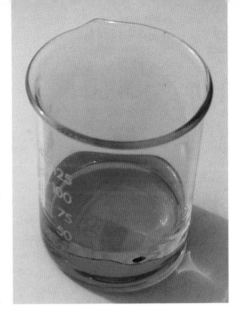

**Ulcerations**
**Splintering pains**
**Chronic catarrh of the mucous membranes**

## Cutaneous disorders:
**Eczema** with fissures and **cracks with clear margins** with blood in the center.
Yellowish plantar warts.

## Digestive disorders:
**Diarrheic stools, intense tenesmus, splintering pains,** mucus and blood.
Anal fissures.
Oral aphthosis, fissured perlèche.

## Urogenital disorders:
• In women
Ulceration and polyp of the cervix, condylomata.
**Sanious leukorrhea.**
Intolerance of IUDs.

• In men
All ulcerated lesions bleeding readily.
**Venereal warts.**

## Aggravation:
– from cold,
– from touch,
– from noise.

## Improvement:
– with warmth,
– with passive movement: riding in a car or a plane (without jolts).

# NUX VOMICA

Poison nut
Loganiaceae

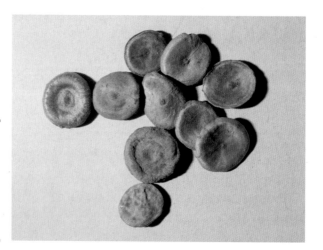

## Disorders linked with a sedentary life
## Hyperexcitability
## Irritability

**Digestive disorders:**
**Desire and abuse of alcoholic drinks and spicy foods, leading to nausea and food vomiting which offers relief.**
The tongue is clear at the front and covered with a whitish coating at the back.
Irresistible **drowsiness after meals,** for about 15 minutes, which facilitates digestion.
Flatulence, constipation, hemorrhoids, headache, migraine.
Motion sickness nausea.

**ENT disorders:**
**Spasmodic rhinitis with sneezing in bouts** as soon as the person gets out of bed.
Coryza caused by cold (after going to the hairdresser).

**Psychological disorders:**
**Nux vomica** is the medicine for overworked businessmen or businesswomen.
Personality disorders, irritability, aggressiveness.
Insomnia with waking up at 3 a.m.

**Aggravation:**
– from alcohol, tobacco, stimulants;
– from medication;
– on waking;
– from cold, drafts.

**Improvement:**
– after a short nap;
– by induced vomiting;
– with warmth.

**Nux vomica** can be used preventively before a good meal (one dose in 12C) or before a surgical intervention under general anesthesia to protect the liver (5 pellets in 12C three or four days before the intervention and also after).

# PETROLEUM

Kerosene

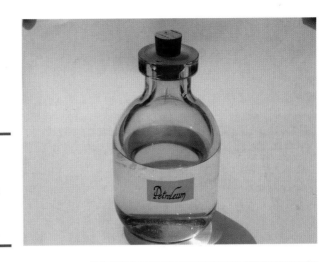

**Winter periodicity and alternation of symptoms between skin and mucous membranes**

**Cutaneous disorders:**
**Cracks and fissures at the tip of the fingers with a dirty aspect.**
Fissured burning chilblains.
Dermatosis caused by hydrocarbons and derivatives.
Oozing vesicular eruptions.

**Digestive disorders:**
**Diarrhea only during the day,** caused by cabbage and sauerkraut or occurring **after an eruption is finished.**

**Motion sickness:**
**Malaise, nausea** improved by eating beforehand or by closing the eyes.

Aggravation:
– from cabbage, sauerkraut;
– in winter;
– in a car, plane, boat.

Improvement:
– in summer,
– with warmth.

# PHOSPHORUS

White phosphorus

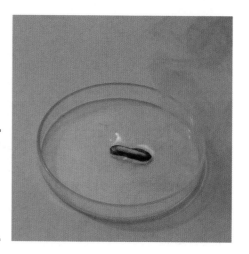

**Alternation between phases of sensorial and intellectual excitation and depressive manifestations with shyness and acute anxiety**

## Hemorrhages:
**Frequent and profuse hemorrhages.**
Epistaxis, digestive hemorrhages, hematuria.
Hemorrhages of wounds and ulcers.
**Preventively** for hemorrhages caused by surgery, dental extraction.

## ENT disorders:
Laryngitis due to vocal straining, with the slightest cold.
Very painful dry cough.
Aphonia with burning pain.

## Digestive disorders:
**Viral hepatitis.**
Pancreatitis.
Cyclic vomiting.

Aggravation:
– from strong emotions, overwork;
– from storms, cold.

Improvement:
– with sleep,
– when eating.

# PHYTOLACCA DECANDRA

Poke
Phytolaccaceae

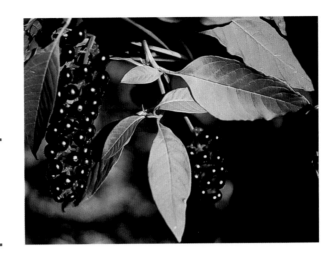

**Dark red tonsillitis**
**Flashing pains**
**Mammary glands**

## ENT disorders:
**Sore throat -** Tonsillitis.
Pharyngitis with burning pain radiating to the ears and neck.
**Deep red mucous membranes.**

## Mammary disorders:
**Mammary dystrophy with cysts.**
Mammary tension and congestion before menses.
Painful mammary engorgement during breast-feeding.
Fissure of the nipple after breast-feeding.

## Pains:
Flashing rheumatic and osseous pains (like electric shocks).
Scapulohumeral periarthritis.

Blepharitis, styes, chalazia.

Aggravation:
— from humidity,
— from cold,
— from movement.

Improvement:
— with dry weather,
— with rest.

# PLATINUM METALLICUM

Platinum

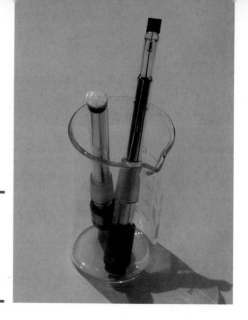

**High opinion of oneself**
**Proud and scornful character**

**Neurological disorders:**
Intestinal **spasms** (sudden onset and end), blepharospasm.
Cramps.
Facial neuralgia.
Headache.

**Gynecological disorders:**
Genital hyperesthesia to touch (medical examination); very painful sexual intercourse.
Hyperestrogenism syndromes.
Excessive libido.

**Digestive disorders:**
Constipation when traveling.

Aggravation:
– from touch, pressure.

Improvement:
– in the open air.

# PLUMBUM METALLICUM

Lead

**Constipation
Sclerosis**

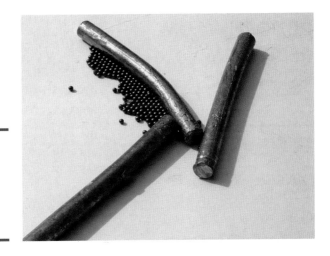

**Digestive disorders:**
**Constipation,** anal spasm with small, hard, black stools (like sheep droppings).
Cramping abdominal pain.
**Violent cramping colic.**

**Sclerosis:**
Cerebral vascular sclerosis.
Loss of memory, behavioral disorders.
Intellectual deficiency; the person fails to understand and trembles.

Anemia.
Optic neuritis.

**Aggravation:**
– in the evening and at night,
– from movement.

**Improvement:**
– with strong pressure,
– when bending double.

# PODOPHYLLUM PELTATUM

May apple
Berberidaceae

## Diarrhea

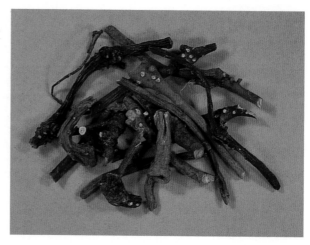

**Diarrhea in children** (especially during teething) **and in adults** (excessive consumption of fresh fruit).
Profuse, watery diarrhea, preceded by rumbling and followed by sensation of abdominal emptiness. This diarrhea is worse in the morning. Abdominal pains relieved when lying prone.

Aggravation:
– early in the morning,
– in hot weather.

Improvement:
– when lying prone.

# PRUNUS SPINOSA

Blackthorn
Rosaceae

## Ocular pains

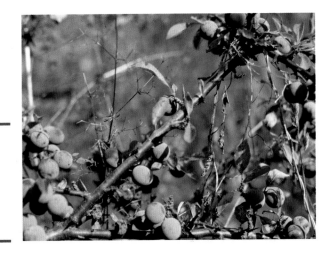

Pain in the eyeball (bursting pains).
Glaucoma.
Ciliary neuralgia.

Ophthalmic zoster.

**Aggravation:**
– from pressure,
– from movement.

**Improvement:**
– when bending over double.

# PULSATILLA

Wind flower
Ranunculaceae

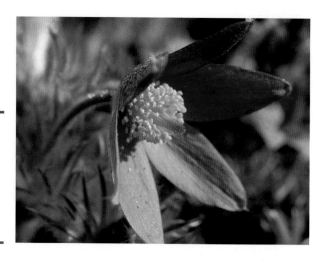

**Great variability of symptoms**
**Aggravated in confined air**
**Acrocyanosis of the extremities**

## Respiratory disorders:
**Rhinitis with nose obstructed at night,** fluent during the day, loss of taste and smell.
Allergic rhinitis.
Dry cough at night, productive during the day;

## Gynecological disorders:
**Long intervals between menses which are scanty and short,** with black blood, flowing especially during the day, and much less at night.
Excessively profuse milk secretion after delivery.

## Circulatory disorders:
**Dilated veins, edema with heat, with immobility.**
Varicose veins, varicose ulcers.
**Cold extremities, icy sensation in cold weather, chilblains.**

## Psychological disorders:
Variability of mood, shifts readily from laughter to tears.
**Improvement with consolation.**
Shyness, blushes readily.

## Infectious diseases:
Measles, rubella.
Mumps.

## Digestive disorders:
**Diarrhea with stools of variable consistency.**
**Loathing and intolerance of greasy foods.**
Craving and intolerance of ice-creams, cakes.
Variable stools (consistency, color).

Aggravation:
— from warmth,
— from rest,
— from ingesting fat,
— from ingesting sugar.

Improvement:
— with fresh air,
— with slow movement,
— with consolation.

# PUTRESCINUM

Putrescine
or tetramethylenediamine
"Super **Pyrogenium**"

---

**Dental infections in particular**

---

....................................................

# PYROGENIUM

Strain of animal origin, autolysate of
muscular tissue
Nosode

---

**Acute or chronic infectious
conditions**

---

Abscesses, furuncles.
Infected wounds.
Dental infections.

Risk of infection with burns.
**Chronic suppuration** (with **Silicea**).

# RANUNCULUS BULBOSUS

Buttercup
Ranunculaceae

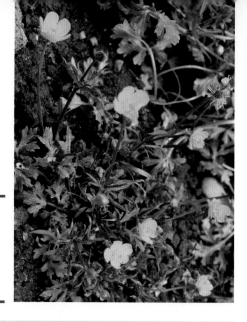

## Intercostal neuralgia and herpes zoster

**especially intercostal herpes zoster and ophthalmic zoster**

Herpes and all vesicular skin diseases containing a bluish liquid with burning pruritus.

Allergic coryza with pruritus in the nostrils.

Aggravation:
– from light touch,
– from changes in the weather.

# RAPHANUS SATIVUS

Black radish
Cruciferae

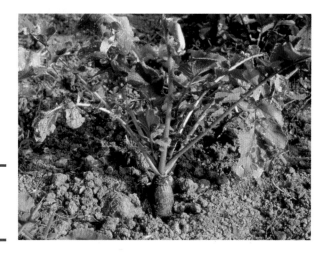

## Abdominal tympanites

**Abdominal tympanites** of patients after surgery, with postoperative interruption of bowel movement.

Constipation with marked global tympanites causing pains relieved by passing wind.

# RHEUM OFFICINALE

Rhubarb
Polygonaceae

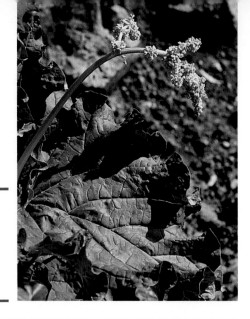

**Diarrhea**

| Diarrhea during teething in infants, brown, clay-like. | Diarrhea following ingestion of unripe fruit (plums). |

**Aggravation:**
– from unripe fruit.

**Improvement:**
– with warmth,
– when bending double.

# RHODODENDRON CHRYSANTHUM

Golden-flowered rhododendron
Ericaceae

## Rheumatic pains

Rheumatic pains and neuralgia starting before a storm, improved afterwards.

Inflammation of the testicles.

Aggravation:
– before a storm.

Improvement:
– after the storm.

# RHUS TOXICODENDRON

Poison ivy
Anacardiaceae

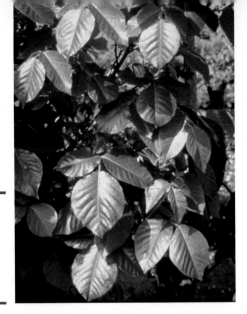

**Erythematous
eruptions
Articular stiffness**

## Cutaneous disorders:
**Vesicular dermatosis,** eczema, herpes, acne, and all types of erythematous and edematous dermatosis improved by applications of very hot water and not relieved by scratching.
Chilblains with itching.
Herpes simplex.

## Febrile conditions:
**High and continuous fever; intense thirst.** Influenza and influenzal conditions with tenderness and need to constantly shift position.

## Muscular disorders:
**Rheumatism or osteoarthritis** aggravated by damp and cold weather, pains with morning stiffness, improved by movement and aggravated at the end of the day.
After muscular effort: sprain, dislocation, sciatica with tearing pains improved by movement.

## ENT disorders:
Hoarseness or coryza after getting wet. **Morning hoarseness with progressive improvement; aggravation towards the end of the day.**

## Aggravation:
– from humidity,
– from immobility,
– from physical fatigue.

## Improvement:
– by changing position,
– with warmth,
– with applications of warm water.

# RICINUS COMMUNIS

Castor bean
Euphorbiaceae

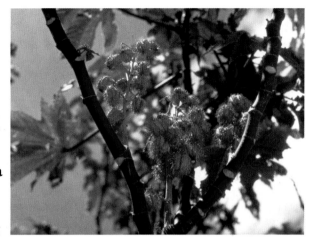

## Choleriform diarrhea
## Breast-feeding

**Choleriform diarrhea** with dehydration.

**Insufficient milk secretion** (in low dilutions 5C, 5 pellets morning and evening).

**To stop milk secretion:** 1 dose in 30C on 3 consecutive mornings.

---

# ROBINIA PSEUDO ACACIA

Black locust
Leguminosae

## Gastralgia
## Migraine
## Hiatal hernia
## Gastroesophageal reflux

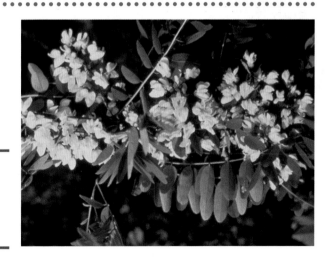

**Gastroesophageal reflux**, hiatal hernia (reflux from gastric hypersecretion).

Nocturnal acidic gastralgia, pyrosis. Migraine with gastric hyperacidity.

# RUMEX CRISPUS

Yellow dock
Polygonaceae

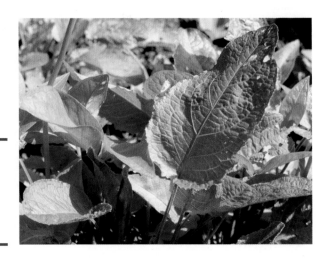

**Disorders triggered
by cold air**

**ENT disorders:**
**Cough triggered by cool air.**
Dry painful cough, with itching in the depression above the sternum.
Sometimes urinary incontinence when coughing.

**Intestinal disorders:**
**Urgent morning diarrhea,** often accompanied by cough.

**Cutaneous disorders:**
Pruritus when undressing, especially of the lower limbs, with eruption or not.

Aggravation:
– from inhaling cool air,
– around 5 a.m.,
– from cold.

Improvement:
– with warmth.

# RUTA GRAVEOLENS

Rue
Rutaceae

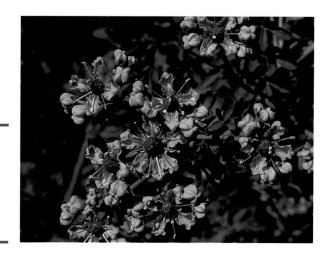

**Traumata**
**Problems of**
**accomodation**

**Traumata:**
Sprain, dislocation, tendinitis, synovial cysts in the wrist, general aching after overexertion or traumatism, or of rheumatic origin. Traumatism of the coccyx.

**Ophthalmology:**
Ocular pains due to straining or to poor lighting (fatigue due to working at a computer screen).

**Aggravation:**
– in cold damp weather,
– from rest.

**Improvement:**
– with movement,
– with warmth.

# SABADILLA

Cevadilla
Liliaceae

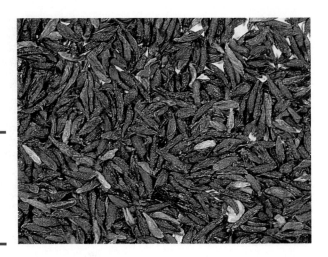

## Spasmodic coryza and hypersensitivity of smell

**Coryza with pronounced spasmodic sneezing,** sensation of burning of the nostrils and **itching of the soft palate,** relieved by applying the tongue.
Hypersensitivity to odor of flowers, fruit, and garlic.

Digestive disorders as a result of parasitosis.

Sensation of having a deformed body (cenesthopathy).

Aggravation:
– from cold,
– from odors (flowers),
– with the full moon and the new moon.

Improvement:
– with warmth,
– with warm drinks.

# SAMBUCUS NIGRA

European elder
Caprifoliaceae

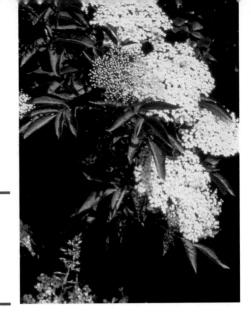

**Coryza**
**Laryngitis stridulosa**

**Dry coryza with total nasal obstruction** compelling the patient to breathe through the mouth.

Children wake up suddenly around midnight with intense suffocation, coughing, dyspnea **(laryngitis stridulosa),** improvement when sitting.

Aggravation:
– at night,
– with the head low.

# SANGUINARIA CANADENSIS

Bloodroot
Papaveraceae

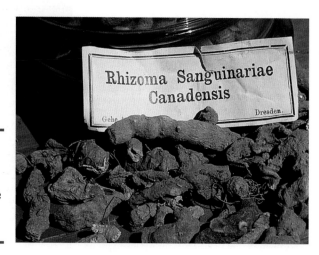

## Periodic and congestive headache

**Circulatory disorders:**
**Periodic migraine** at the week-end. Throbbing, congestive headache (menopause).
**Hot flushes of menopause,** limited to the cheeks and ears, hot flushes of hypertensive patients and alcoholics. Intense burning of the palms of the hands and feet.

**Respiratory disorders:**
**Spasmodic coryza with hypersensitivity to flower odors,** irritant discharge of the nostrils, sneezing. Polyps of the nose with tendency to bleeding.
Dry cough with burning of the trachea.

**Aggravation:**
– from noise, odors, movement, light (circulatory disorders);
– from odor of flowers.

**Improvement:**
– with sleep.

# SEPIA

Cuttlefish ink
Sepiidae

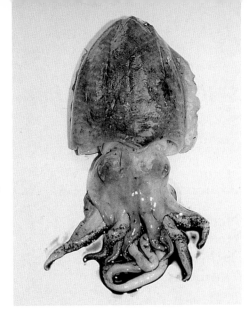

**Depression**
**Stasis**
**Ptosis**

## Behavioral disorders:
Reactive depressive condition with **pessimism**, discouragement, **indifference** to family and work.
Very intense fatigue, especially in the morning.
**Seeks solitude, cannot bear consolation**, generally negative outlook.

## Urogenital disorders:
Sensation of pelvic and genital heaviness, frequent urge to urinate.
Irritant chronic leukorrhea.
Aversion for any form of sexual activity.
Recurrent urinary infections.

## Cutaneous disorders:
Ageing of the skin with yellowish stains.

Genital herpes or herpes simplex.
Mycotic eczema.
Fissural psoriasis.

## Digestive disorders:
**Disgust for food** and milk which causes diarrhea; **desire of vinegar, pickles, acidic and highly-flavored foods.**
Uncontrollable vomiting, **hypersensitivity to cooking odors.**
Sensation of gastric emptiness or of abdominal heaviness.
Constipation, sensation of rectal fullness, hemorrhoids.
**Migraine.**
Nausea during the first months of **pregnancy,** frequent presence of mask of pregnancy.

Aggravation:
– from cold,
– from standing,
– from consolation.

Improvement:
– with energetic exercising (dancing),
– with warmth.

# SPIGELIA ANTHELMIA

Pink root
Loganiaceae

---

**Migraine**
**Neuralgia**
**Tachycardia**
**Pinworms**

---

### Migraine and neuralgia:
**Ophthalmic migraine,** frontal and occipital first, above the left orbit subsequently.
**Neuralgia** with violent tearing pains of the trigeminal nerve, **postherpetic neuralgia,** intense ocular pain.

### Tachycardia:
**Palpitations, angina pectoris,** cardiac pain radiating to the left arm.

### Pinworms:
Pale face, bad breath, headache, palpitations.

Aggravation:
– from touch,
– from movement,
– from cold air (neuralgia).

Improvement:
– with rest,
– when lying on the right-hand side.

# SPONGIA TOSTA

Roasted sponge
Euspongia

## Dyspnea and laryngeal coughing

The person wakes up suddenly before midnight with dyspnea and acute anxiety ("breathing as if through a sponge").
**Laryngitis** with characteristic cough resembling the sound of a saw cutting through a pine-wood board.

**Laryngitis stridulosa.**
Hoarseness with dryness of the pharynx and vocal cords, burning pains when speaking.

Aggravation:
– around midnight,
– when lying with the head low.

Improvement:
– with warm drinks,
– when lying with the head high up.

# STAPHYSAGRIA

Stavesacre
Ranunculaceae

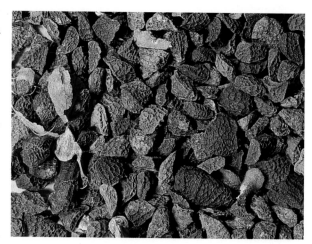

**Neurosis**
**Pruritus**
**Styes**
**Chalazia**
**Cystitis**

Repressed hypersensitivity.

**Psychological disorders:**
Psychological disorders, depression, **neurosis after humiliation,** indignation, injustice (real or felt), extreme touchiness.

**Cutaneous disorders:**
**Pruritus changing place** after scratching.

Postoperative pain of clean surgical **wounds** (scalpel).
**Chalazia, recurrent styes.**

**Urogenital disorders:**
**Cystalgia with clear urine.**
Cystitis in the newly-wed.
Urinary disorders of difficult pregnancy.

Aggravation:
– from indignation, anger, humiliation;
– from the slightest touch on the
  affected areas.

# STICTA PULMONARIA

Lungwort
Stictaceae

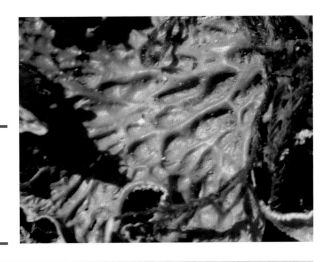

**Coryza**
**Nasal obstruction**
**Dry cough**

**ENT disorders:**
Acute or chronic, or allergic **coryza**, with **nasal obstruction**, painful at the root of the nose, sensation of heaviness at the root of the nose, dryness of the mucosa, retrosternal discharge.

**Dry cough,** irritant, unremitting, mainly at night with pains in the frontal sinuses when breathing in.

Improvement:
– from nasal discharge.

# SYMPHORI-CARPUS RACEMOSUS

Snowberry
Caprifoliaceae

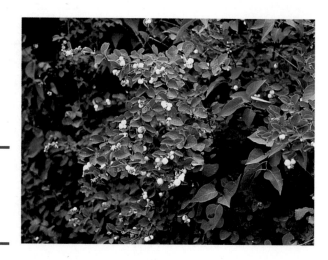

**Nausea**
**Vomiting**

**Nausea and vomiting** aggravated with the slightest movement.

Persistent vomiting of pregnancy with aversion for food.

Aggravation:
– from the slightest movement.

Improvement:
– with rest.

# SYMPHYTUM OFFICINALE

Comfrey
Boraginaceae

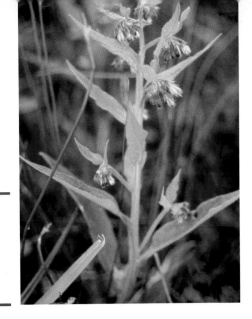

## Traumatism of the bones

| Traumatism of the bones and of the periosteum. | Consolidation of fractures. |
|---|---|
| | Sequelae of traumatism of the eye-balls. |

# TABACUM

Tobacco
Solanaceae

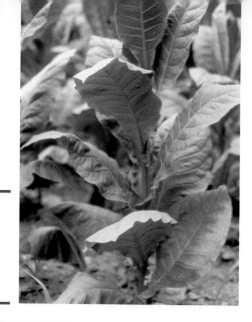

## Motion sickness

**Nausea, vomiting;** condition aggravated by the slightest movement, improved in the open air, when closing the eyes. Pale face, weakness, icy cold skin.

Vomiting of pregnancy with hypersalivation.

Aggravation:
– in a warm room,
– from movement.

Improvement:
– in the open air.

# TARENTULA CUBENSIS

Tarantula
Lycosidae

---

**Insect bites
and stings
Agitation**

---

**Deep red tissue inflammation** with induration (spider bites); also furuncles, abscesses.

**Agitation,** instability, sleeping disorders, improved by music.

Aggravation:
– from touch,
– from light,
– from movement.

Improvement:
– with music,
– in the open air.

# THUJA OCCIDENTALIS

White cedar
Cupressaceae

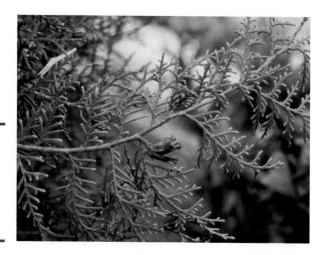

## Warts
## Cellulitis

**Chronic genital infection**
**Prevention of complications of vaccination**

### Warts:
**Thuja occidentalis** is the major medicine for warts. To be given whatever the location and aspect of the wart, 1 unit-dose a week in 30C. Complement with **Dulcamara, Antimonium crudum**, etc.

Locally, **Thuja occidentalis** ointment on warts, cystic and pustular acne, papillomas, condylomata.

### Cellulitis:
Tendency to adipose cellular imbibition of tissues. 1 dose per week in 9C.

### Genital disorders:
Purulent leukorrhea.
Fibromas, polyps, ovarian cysts.

### Prevention of complications of vaccinations:
1 unit-dose in 9C before the vaccination, in combination with 1 dose of **Sulphur 9C**, 48 hours after the vaccination.

### Aggravation:
— from damp cold,
— from vaccinations.

### Improvement:
— with dry warmth,
— when stretching.

# URTICA URENS

Dwarf nettle
Urticaceae

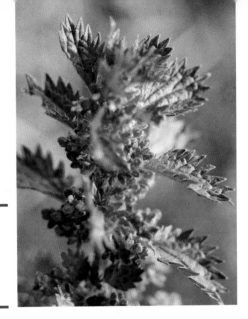

## Urticaria (with pruritus)
## Gout

**Urticaria with pruritus,** burning, sting or bite, aggravated by contact with cold water.

Acute gout, alternating gout and urticaria.

**Aggravation:**
– from contact with water.

# VERATRUM ALBUM

White hellebore
Liliaceae

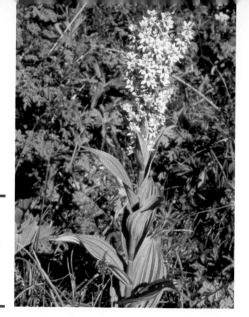

**Exhaustion with cold sweating, vomiting, diarrhea, prostration**

### Digestive disorders:
**Choleriform spurting diarrhea, profuse,** urgent, with loss of facial color, **cold sweating** and cramping pains, violent vomiting.

### Gynecological disorders:
**Dysmenorrhea with hemorrhagic menses,** vomiting, exhaustion, cold sweating, cramping pains.

### Aggravation:
– in damp cold weather,
– from movement

### Improvement:
– with warmth.

# VIPERA BERUS

Asp
Viperidae

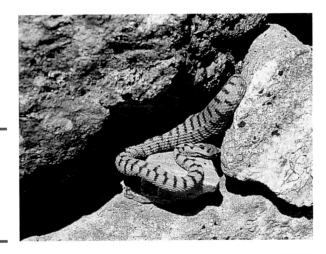

**Phlebitis
Varicose veins**

| Superficial phlebitis. | Varicose veins, feeling of heaviness in the legs with bursting pains. |

**Aggravation:**
– when letting the legs dangle.

**Improvement:**
– when keeping the legs raised.

# ZINCUM METALLICUM

Zinc

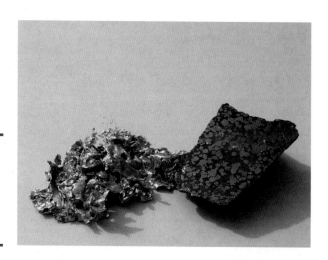

**Asthenia
Restless legs**

**Psychological and nervous asthenia,** exhaustion, dejection, depression.
**Slowness of comprehension** (repeats question before answering them).
Problems at school or intellectual overexertion resulting in memory disorders.

**Dysmenorrhea** with painful premenstrual syndrome, improved by discharge.

**"Restless legs" syndrome.**
Anorexia or dyspepsia with intolerance of wine.
Alternation between dermatosis and neuralgic syndrome.
**Herpes zoster when the eruption has difficulty breaking out.**

Aggravation:
– from wine,
– from noise,
– from touch,
– from the disappearance of an eruption or a normal elimination.

Improvement:
– with a physiological discharge,
– with a cutaneous eruption.

# INDEX

# M

malaria 169
mammary dystrophy 156, 217
mammary engorgement 217
mammary glands, disorders 217
mastoiditis 161
measles 222
memory disturbances 142, 195
memory, loss of 182, 219
menometrorrhagia 169
menopause, hot flushes 92, 153, 183, 199, 234
menses, hemorrhagic 209
menses, interrupted 199
menses, long intervals between m. 222
menses, painful m. with cramps 163
metrorrhagia 199
migraine 198, 214, 229, 234, 235
migraine, ophthalmic 193, 236
milk crusts 157
motion sickness 98, 155, 170, 214, 215, 242
mucous membranes, burning 164
mucous membranes, dryness 153, 156
mucus, abundant 146
mucus, thick whitish 197
mumps 206, 222
mycosis 209

# N

nausea 187, 214, 215, 240, 242
nausea, during menses 170
nausea, odor 190
nausea, pregnancy 105, 235
nausea, violent 192
necrosis, maxillary 188
nephritis 147, 160
nerve endings, pains 189
nervous anticipation 148, 182
neuralgia 138, 140, 150, 175, 203, 227, 236
neuralgia, cervical 200
neuralgia, dental 165
neuralgia, facial 204, 208, 218
neuralgia, intercostal 208, 224
neuralgia, trigeminal 172
neuritis, optic 219

neuritis, stumps 140
neuromuscular disorders 167
neurosis 238
nipple, crack 162
nipple, fissure 184, 217
nose, obstruction 202, 233, 239
nosebleed 78
nutrition, disorders 157, 211

# O

obesity 157
osteitis 185
osteoarthritis 185, 228
osteoporosis 158, 188
otitis 100, 138, 150, 165
otitis, congestive 153, 161, 180
ovarialgia 198
overeating 145, 157
overexertion 149, 231
overweight 157

# P

pain, absence of 158
pain, acute shooting 203
pain, bending double 203
pain, burning 150, 160, 188, 206, 216, 217, 237
pain, cervical 167, 200
pain, eye 147, 231, 236
pain, eyeballs 178, 221
pain, flashing 217
pain, in localized points 156
pain, influenza 178
pain, intolerance 165
pain, menstrual 163
pain, nerve endings 189
pain, rheumatic 108, 147, 177, 217, 227
pain, splintering 186, 213
pain, visceral 175
pains and aches 182
pallor, marked 146
palpitations 236
pancreatitis 216
paralysis 164
paralysis of vocal cords 164
paralysis, facial 164

PHOTOGRAPHIC CREDITS

Professor Jacques Pellecuer, Faculty of Pharmacy, University of Montpellier:
p.138, 139d, 152, 160, 163, 167, 168, 169, 170, 173u, 173d,
182, 187, 192, 217, 220, 232, 234, 238

Promonature 71 Briant:
p. 209, 240, 247

Ecole Normale Supérieure de Lyon – Laboratoire des Sciences de la Terre:
p. 142, 143, 146, 150, 155, 174, 184, 188, 195, 196, 197, 204, 205l, 205r,
206, 213, 215, 216, 218, 219, 248

Boiron – Botany Laboratory:
all other photographs

Achevé d'imprimer sous les presses de l'imprimerie Brailly – France
Juin 2008